Basic Psychological Insights for Psychotherapy

Rainer Sachse

Basic Psychological Insights for Psychotherapy

How an Integrative Approach to Psychotherapy Can Succeed

Springer

Rainer Sachse
IPP Bochum
Bochum, Nordrhein-Westfalen
Germany

ISBN 978-3-662-69779-5 ISBN 978-3-662-69780-1 (eBook)
https://doi.org/10.1007/978-3-662-69780-1

Translation from the German language edition: "Psychologische Grunderkenntnisse für Psychotherapie" by Rainer Sachse, © Der/die Herausgeber bzw. der/die Autor(en), exklusiv lizenziert an Springer-Verlag GmbH, DE, ein Teil von Springer Nature 2023. Published by Springer Berlin Heidelberg. All Rights Reserved.

This book is a translation of the original German edition "Psychologische Grunderkenntnisse für Psychotherapie" by Rainer Sachse, published by Springer-Verlag GmbH, DE in 2023. The translation was done with the help of an artificial intelligence machine translation tool. A subsequent human revision was done primarily in terms of content, so that the book will read stylistically differently from a conventional translation. Springer Nature works continuously to further the development of tools for the production of books and on the related technologies to support the authors.

This Springer imprint is published by the registered company Springer-Verlag GmbH, DE, part of Springer Nature.
The registered company address is: Heidelberger Platz 3, 14197 Berlin, Germany

Contents

About the Author

Prof. Dr. Rainer Sachse is a graduate psychologist, psychological psychotherapist, founder of "Clarification-Oriented Psychotherapy" and head of the Institute for Psychological Psychotherapy (IPP) in Bochum; his main areas of work are personality styles and personality disorders. He has written numerous books on psychotherapy and personality disorders, including some satirical guides on how to ruin your relationship, your career, and your life. Rainer Sachse presents complex psychological facts in a generally understandable way and portrays them humorously and empathetically.

1

Introduction: Purpose of the Book

The aim of the book is to reflect on the general principles that can be derived from psychology for a conception of psychotherapy that should be considered in the theory and practice of therapy.

The considerations are derived from various sources: from theory and research in psychology, from psychotherapy research, but also from many years of experience in psychotherapy, supervision, and training.

Such considerations should be made that are *cross-conceptual*, i.e., not specifically related to a particular form of therapy, but can indeed be considered as overarching.

A key goal of this approach is to create a basis for further reflection on psychotherapy, both in terms of theoretical concepts and practical procedures.

Different aspects should become clear:

- that it makes sense to take psychological theories and research more into account in the conception of psychotherapy;
- that we should move away from very limited models and theories;
- i.e., while it is very sensible to develop specific theories and procedures for specific disorders,
- these "special therapies" should be embedded in an *overarching conception* of psychotherapy, e.g., to make procedures more compatible and more comprehensively substantiated;
- that it should be clearly recognized that "special therapies" require specific theoretical concepts and procedures, but such therapies are not identical

R. Sachse, *Basic Psychological Insights for Psychotherapy*,
https://doi.org/10.1007/978-3-662-69780-1_1

with "*the* psychotherapies": that the results of specific procedures for specific disorders and clients can *just* ***not*** be generalized and transferred to other disorders and clients; one cannot consider a part of psychotherapy as *the* psychotherapy. This should be clearly recognized and taken into account, and an overarching conception helps with this. This results in,

- that not only very specific strategies should be developed, but psychotherapy should be broadened to be able to embed individual procedures *into a framework concept;*
- that because of the grounding of psychotherapy in psychology, it is also necessary to create a "psychological identity" of psychotherapy, i.e., to decide which type of concepts, terminologies, etc. one wants to integrate and which not;
- that the extreme heterogeneity of clients (but also of therapists and therapies) should definitely be taken into account, which implies,
- that therapies should be created that fit *clients*, not just "symptoms";
- that it should be seen that psychotherapy is *a service for clients*, that one should therefore analyze what clients really need and want and that one should not be therapy-centered, i.e., only offer clients those procedures that are currently "in", and also not therapist-centered, i.e., only offer such therapy that suits one as a therapist, but that one ensures that clients really get what they need; and that this means,
- that psychotherapy should essentially be *client-centered*, not in an ideological, but in a psychological sense;
- that psychotherapy must be seen as a *complex procedure*, in which complex initial conditions of clients, therapy processes, etc. should be taken into account and that this requires a (very) high expertise of therapists.

Some aspects will be discussed here that can be considered particularly *central*, but this does not mean that this list is complete or that other aspects are irrelevant.

Part 1 of the book will address some basic questions about therapy conception.

Part 2 will discuss some practical problems and procedures in psychotherapy.

Part 3 will discuss some basic problems of clients to show which psychological aspects therapists should pay attention to and which (process) goals they can sensibly pursue.

Part I

Basic Considerations on Psychotherapy

In this section, some basic considerations for a conception of psychotherapy will be made. This is also intended to draw attention to some "misconceptions" about psychotherapy.

2

Why is a Client a Client?

This chapter is about reflecting on what it psychologically means for a person to be a client and what psychotherapeutic implications are associated with it, which must be taken into account in psychotherapy.

An important question, the answer to which has central implications for a conception of psychotherapy, is why a client is a client at all, why he therefore seeks a psychotherapist.

Obviously, a client becomes a client,

- because he has psychological problems,
- which cause him costs that he does not want,
- which he cannot solve (well enough) on his own,
- which he cannot solve even with the help of his context (partner, friends etc.),
- for the processing of which he therefore wants to seek professional help.

This implies:

- A client has psychological problems: He has certain symptoms, crises, conflicts, i.e., a kind of problems that can be described psychologically and that can be addressed psychotherapeutically. *Otherwise, psychotherapy would not be indicated at all.*

R. Sachse, *Basic Psychological Insights for Psychotherapy*,
https://doi.org/10.1007/978-3-662-69780-1_2

- The client recognizes that the problems cause him personal costs (conflicts, restrictions, dissatisfaction, health problems, etc.) *and*
- the client has realized that he cannot solve the problems adequately and cannot receive effective help from his context either. This makes him *motivated for therapy.*
- He seeks an expert to effectively help him solve his problems, i.e., *he expects effective assistance.*
- This also implies that the problem is apparently so complex or so constituted that professional help seems necessary.

The reasons why the client cannot solve a problem on his own can be varied:

- A significant reason lies in the *limited processing capacities* of humans. If a problem is complex in itself, it already requires a high degree of capacity to consider, clarify, understand it, i.e., the consideration of the problem-*contents* is very complex.
- The problem must then also be constructively processed, which implies,
  - developing questions,
  - following questions,
  - controlling and monitoring clarification processes,
  - deliberately questioning schemas etc.

  and all this requires even more capacity.

Given the limited processing capacity of humans, such tasks are *not manageable* for *one person.* This aspect of a human's limited processing capacity is also of central importance for the conception of psychotherapy and for the definition of expertise (see Baddeley, 2010; Cowan, 2001, 2010; Klingberg, 2000, 2009; Logie, 2011; Marois & Ivanoff, 2005).

Thus, a person alone is *necessarily overwhelmed:* This is the reason why therapy requires *two* people:

- The client as the *expert for the contents and*
- the therapist as the *expert for the process.*
- To effectively solve certain types of problems, the therapist needs a *know-how:* One must know how to proceed, what to do when, etc. (see Sachse, 1991a, 1992a, b, c).

- This *expertise* has developed therapy concepts and therapy research. Even psychotherapists struggle and take a long time to acquire such expertise.

Logically, a client cannot even begin to possess such expertise. Therefore, he cannot solve his problem simply because he does not have the necessary know-how!

- Clients *"are also stuck in biased processing":* They make false assumptions, use incorrect models and thus incorrect approaches to solutions, keep asking the same (wrong) questions, do "more of the same" etc. They have developed solutions that they stick to, but these do not solve the problem, but may even exacerbate it ("I have a solution, but unfortunately it does not fit my problem"). And that's why they *absolutely* need a therapist, *who controls their processing processes,* who conveys effective approaches and prevents wrong procedures (cf. Gäßler & Sachse, 1992a, b; Sachse, 1984, 1986, 1988, 1990a, b, c, 1991a, b, 1992a, d).
- Some of their problems, schemas, etc. are (strongly) aversive or self-esteem burdening. Thus, they *avoid* systematically dealing with these aspects (cf. Sachse, 2003, 2008, 2016; Sachse et al. 2011).

However, psychologically it is true: *Any kind of avoidance preserves a problem!* Clients can (e.g. due to manipulations) derive benefits from their problems, so they are ambivalent: They want to get rid of the "costs", but keep the benefits. They are therefore not really *motivated to change.* Therefore, they need a therapist who confronts them with this and shows them *that* they are ambivalent.

So, psychologically, it is not surprising that people often cannot solve (complex) problems themselves effectively: This is normal and to be expected. But this does not mean in any way that disorders are "psychopathological": They are rather an aspect of normal psychology: As Fiedler (2003, 2007) says, they are "extreme variants of normal psychological functioning".

And therefore, it cannot be dishonorable in any way to seek a therapist! On the contrary, it is extremely sensible!

So there are several basic psychological insights:

- *If I do not perceive relevant aspects of the problem, I cannot understand them and thus the problem.*
- And a problem that I do not understand, I cannot solve.
- Because even relatively simple problems can no longer be solved by "trial and error": One must know how the problem "works" in order to find effective solutions.

This makes it clear once again,

- Clients are clients because they cannot solve problems themselves,
- they come to psychotherapy because they need professional help,
- a therapist must *specifically help* them and therefore he must do different things than clients usually experience in everyday life,
- a therapist needs high expertise for effective help.

> This means: *A client must have different and more constructive experiences in psychotherapy than in everyday life.*

Otherwise, the therapy will be as effective as everyday life, namely *not at all.*

And: The client should not have any experiences, but those that specifically help him solve the problem! The therapeutic offer must therefore fit the problem as closely as possible.

Therefore, it makes little sense to deal with the previous, failed solutions in therapy: Since they have obviously proven to be ineffective, this is a waste of time.

Therefore, it is necessary for the therapist and client to analyze the problem very thoroughly once again psychologically *and then* develop new approaches to solutions.

As we will see, however, one must fundamentally distinguish between *therapy motivation* and *change motivation*: Therapy motivation is the motivation to enter therapy, change motivation is the decision to actively change something.

Here, therefore, only therapy motivation is discussed (see Sachse, 2009, 2015; Sachse & Langens, 2015; Sachse et al., 2012, 2018)!

This has some implications for psychotherapy:

- Therapists must take on a specific task in the process.
- They thus assume *process responsibility.*
- They must develop the necessary expertise.
- And they must use this specifically.

References

Baddeley, A. D. (2010). *Working memory. Current biology, 20*(4), 136–140.

Cowan, N. (2001). The magical number 4 in short-term memory: A reconsideration of mental storage capacity. *Behavioural Brain Science, 24*(1), 87–114.

Cowan, N. (2010). The magical mystery four: How is working memory capacity limited, and why? *Current directions in psychological science, 19*(1), 51–57.

Fiedler, P. (2003). *Integrative Psychotherapie bei Persönlichkeitsstörungen* (2nd edn.). Hogrefe.

Fiedler, P. (2007). *Persönlichkeitsstörungen* (6th edn.). Beltz.

Gäßler, B., & Sachse, R. (1992a). Psychotherapeuten als Experten: Unter welchen Voraussetzungen können Psychotherapeuten die komplexe sprachliche Information ihrer Klienten verarbeiten? In R. Sachse, G., Lietaer, & W. B. Stiles (Eds.), *Neue Handlungskonzepte der Klientenzentrierten Psychotherapie* (pp. 133–142). Asanger.

Gäßler, B., & Sachse, R. (1992b). Psychotherapeuten als Experten. In: L. Montada (Ed.), *Bericht über den 38. Kongress der Deutschen Gesellschaft für Psychologie in Trier, 1,* 663–664. Hogrefe.

Klingberg, T. (2000). Limitations in information processing in the human brain: Neuroimaging of dual task performance and working memory tasks. *Progress in brain research, 126*, 95–102.

Klingberg, T. (2009). *The overflowing brain: Information overload and the limits of working memory*. University Press.

Logie, R. H. (2011). The functional organization and capacity limits of working memory. *Current directions in Psychological Science, 20*(4), 240–245.

Marois, R., & Ivanoff, J. (2005). Capacity limits of information processing in the brain. *Trends in cognitive Sciences, 9*(6), 296–305.

Sachse, R. (1984). Vertiefende Interventionen in der Klientenzentrierten Psychotherapie. *Partnerberatung, 5,* 106–113.

Sachse, R. (1986). Was bedeutet „Selbstexploration" und wie kann ein Therapeut den Selbstklärungsprozeß des Klienten fördern? Versuch einer theoretischen Klärung mit Hilfe sprachpsychologischer Konzepte. *GwG-Info, 64,* 33–52.

Sachse, R. (1988). Das Konzept des empathischen Verstehens: Versuch einer sprachpsychologischen Klärung und Konsequenzen für das therapeutische Handeln. In GwG (Eds.), *Orientierung an der Person: Diesseits und Jenseits von Psychotherapie,* Vol. 2, 162–174. GwG.

Sachse, R. (1990a). Acting purposefully in client-centered therapy. In P. J. D. Drenth, J. A. Sergeant, & R.-J. Takens (Eds.), *European perspectives in psychology, 1* (pp. 65–80). Wiley.

Sachse, R. (1990b). Concrete interventions are crucial: The influence of therapist's processing-proposals on the client's intra-personal exploration. In G. Lietaer, J.

Rombauts, & R. van Balen (Eds.), *Client-centered and experiential psychotherapy in the nineties* (pp. 295–308). University Press.

Sachse, R. (1990c). The influence of therapists' processing proposals on the explication process of the client. *Person-Centered Review, 5,* 321–344.

Sachse, R. (1991a). Zielorientiertes Handeln in der Gesprächspsychotherapie: Steuerung des Explizierungsprozesses von Klienten durch zentrale Bearbeitungsangebote des Therapeuten. In D. Schulte (Eds.), *Therapeutische Entscheidungen* (pp. 89–106). Hogrefe.

Sachse, R. (1991b). Spezifische Wirkfaktoren in der Klientenzentrierten Psychotherapie: Zur Bedeutung von Bearbeitungsangeboten und Inhaltsbezügen. *Verhaltenstherapie und psychosoziale Praxis, 23,* 157–171.

Sachse, R. (1992a). *Zielorientierte Gesprächspsychotherapie – Eine grundlegende Neukonzeption.* Hogrefe.

Sachse, R. (1992b). Psychotherapie als komplexe Aufgabe: Verarbeitungs-, Intentionsbildungs- und Handlungsplanungsprozesse bei Psychotherapeuten. In R. Sachse, G. Lietaer, & W. B. Stiles (Eds.), *Neue Handlungskonzepte der Klientenzentrierten Psychotherapie* (pp. 109–112). Asanger.

Sachse, R. (1992c). Informationsverarbeitungs- und Handlungsplanungsprozesse bei Psychotherapeuten. In: L. Montada (Eds.), *Bericht über den 38. Kongress der Deutschen Gesellschaft für Psychologie in Trier, 2,* 942–946. Hogrefe.

Sachse, R. (1992d). Zielorientiertes Handeln in der Gesprächspsychotherapie: Zum tatsächlichen und notwendigen Einfluß von Therapeuten auf die Explizierungsprozesse bei Klienten. *Zeitschrift für Klinische Psychologie, 21,* 286–301.

Sachse, R. (2003). *Klärungsorientierte Psychotherapie.* Hogrefe.

Sachse, R. (2008). Klärungsprozesse in der Psychotherapie. In J. Margraf & S. Schneider (Eds.), *Lehrbuch der Verhaltenstherapie* (3rd edn., pp. 227–232). Springer.

Sachse, R. (2009). Möglichkeiten und Grenzen der Motivierung von Klienten im Therapieprozess. In M. Saimeh (Eds.), *Motivation und Widerstand* (pp. 116–133). Psychiatrie-Verlag.

Sachse, R. (2015). Änderungs- und Stabilisierungsmotivation in der Therapie und ihre therapeutische Beeinflussung. In: R. Sachse, S. Schirm, & S. Kiszkenow-Bäker (Eds.), *Klärungsorientierte Psychotherapie in der Praxis* (pp. 111–122). Pabst.

Sachse, R. (2016). *Klärungsprozesse in der Klärungsorientierten Psychotherapie.* Hogrefe.

Sachse, R., Fasbender, J., & Sachse, M. (2011). Die Bearbeitung von Vermeidung in der Klärungsorientierten Psychotherapie. In: R. Sachse, J. Fasbender, J. Breil, & M. Sachse (Eds.), *Perspektiven Klärungsorientierter Psychotherapie II* (pp. 156–183). Pabst.

Sachse, R., & Langens, T. A. (2015). Motivierung von Klienten im Therapieprozess: Herstellung und Steigerung von Änderungsmotivation.

In: R. Sachse, S. Schirm, & S. Kiszkenow-Bäker (Eds.), *Klärungsorientierte Psychotherapie in der Praxis* (pp. 97–110). Pabst.

Sachse, R., Langens, T. A., & Sachse, M. (2012). *Klienten motivieren – Therapeutische Strategien zur Stärkung der Änderungsbereitschaft*. Psychiatrie-Verlag.

Sachse, R., Langens, T. A., & Sachse, M. (2018). *Klienten motivieren* (2nd edn.). Psychiatrie-Verlag.

3

Heterogeneity

This chapter explains how extremely heterogeneous clients are at the start of therapy in terms of important psychological variables and what consequences this has for a conception of psychotherapy.

Kiesler (1966a, b, 1969) warned of a "homogeneity myth": the assumption that all clients are the same, that the same therapeutic offer can be made to all clients, that all therapists are the same, and that different forms of therapy work in the same way.

However, the homogeneity myth is widespread in psychotherapy and sometimes leads to clearly false conclusions (cf. Sachse, 2013).

Psychotherapy research has definitively shown that there is an *extremely high degree of heterogeneity* in the field of psychotherapy. Clients show very different "entry characteristics" that they bring to therapy and that influence the therapy outcome and process (e.g., Blatt et al., 1995; DiClemente et al., 1991; Frank, 1974; Jenkins et al., 1986; Michelson & Morley, 1987; Piper et al., 1991, 1992).

This heterogeneity exists on the client side:

- Clients exhibit extremely *different characteristics* that they bring to therapy: personality styles, openness, trust, expectations, etc. These characteristics can all have an impact on psychotherapy: on what clients expect, how they respond to relationship building and interventions, what therapy goals they need, etc.

R. Sachse, *Basic Psychological Insights for Psychotherapy*,
https://doi.org/10.1007/978-3-662-69780-1_3

For a detailed presentation of these aspects, see Sachse (2022).

- The mental problems and disorders are *extremely heterogeneous:* They vary in severity, generate different costs, and above all: *They function psychologically in extremely different ways!*

This makes it clear that

- clients require different, individual case concepts or client models,
- different therapeutic approaches,
- different therapeutic strategies, etc. *are required* (cf. Sachse, 2022).

Therapists are also highly heterogeneous:

- They represent different therapeutic directions.
- They therefore apply very different concepts for modeling the problem.
- They implement very different therapeutic strategies and procedures.
- They show different personality styles, preferences, and biases.
- They have *content-wise* very different expertise, and for this reason, they implement very different procedures.
- But they also differ greatly in the *extent* of their expertise, which strongly influences the quality of their therapeutic work.

This results in some insights:

- *Obviously, not all clients can be treated therapeutically in the same way,* but a therapist must adapt individually to the client.
- He must develop a specific client model and derive strategies, interventions, etc. from it.
- He cannot make the "same relationship offer" to all clients.

Clients bring very different disorders to therapy. And these disorders can function psychologically in different ways (cf. Beckham, 1989; Casper et al., 2008, 2017a, b; Freyberger & Caspar, 2008).

Even if two clients have the same disorder (diagnostically), they can still be highly different in many relevant psychological variables.

Therefore, a pure diagnosis, which always only describes a "symptom surface", can never be sufficient to derive targeted therapeutic interventions and strategies.

In any case, a therapist must work out an individual case concept as a "client model" with the client (cf. Sachse, 2017).

From *this*, indication decisions are then derived.

But not only are clients highly heterogeneous, but so are therapists (e.g. Caspar & Große-Holtforth, 2009; Coady, 1991; Elliott et al., 2008; Greenberg & Safran, 1989; Shaw et al., 1999; Truax & Mitchell, 1971). For a detailed overview, see Sachse (2022).

Therapy processes are highly diverse (see e.g. Barber et al., 2000; Haas et al., 2002; Orlinsky & Howard, 1978, 1986; Orlinsky et al., 1994; Orlinsky et al., 2004). Thus, they are *highly complex.*

Another important conclusion from the strong heterogeneity is *that scientific results cannot be generalized* and if so, only if there are very good reasons for it (see Sachse, 2022):

- Results from one disorder group (e.g. phobias) can never be generalized to other disorder groups (e.g. personality disorders).
  Personality disorders are much more complex disorders that psychologically "function differently" than phobias and therefore require completely different interventions (see Sachse, 2022).
  For example, the result that "standard therapy" can be done with phobic clients based only on diagnoses and individual case concepts are unnecessary, *cannot be transferred to other disorders in any way and especially not generalized for more complex disorders!* Such a generalization is not accurate and leads to completely wrong results, i.e. conclusions that do not apply to the disorder group for which the generalizing assumptions are made.
- From the results obtained with certain therapists, with a certain orientation, expertise, training, etc., no conclusions can be drawn about therapists of other orientations and expertise.
  What therapists can do depends on the type of their training, their expertise, etc.: However, psychotherapy trainings are also highly heterogeneous!
- What therapists of a sample can or cannot do, cannot be inferred to other therapists.
- Results obtained from highly controlled (and thus strongly limited) conditions cannot be readily applied to the highly complex reality of psychotherapy (see Sachse, 2022).

Therefore, scientific findings cannot simply be *"applied"* in practice: Therapeutic practice creates *entirely different contextual conditions,* than research does. Many studies show that results found under controlled conditions often cannot be replicated in the field of practice.

If such generalizations are made, errors are made in inductive conclusions (Popper, 1994, 2005) and implicitly follow a clearly falsified (!!) assumption of homogeneity.

References

Barber, J. P., Connolly, M. B., Crits-Christoph, P., Gladis, L., & Siqueland, L. (2000). Alliance predicts patients' outcomes beyond in-treatment change in symptoms. *Journal of Consulting and Clinical Psychology, 68,* 1027–1032.

Beckham, E. E. (1989). Improvement after evaluation in psychotherapy of depression: Evidence of a placebo effect? *Journal of Clinical Psychology, 45,* 945–950.

Blatt, S. J., Quinlan, D. M., Pilkonis, P. A., & Shea, T. M. (1995). Impact of perfectionism and need for approval on the brief treatment of depression: The national institute of mental health treatment of depression collaborative research program revisited. *Journal of Consulting and Clinical Psychology, 63,* 125–132.

Caspar, F., & Grosse Holtforth, M. (2009). Responsiveness – Eine entscheidende Prozessvariable in der Psychotherapie. *Zeitschrift für Klinische Psychologie und Psychotherapie, 38*(1), 61–69.

Caspar, F., Herpertz, S.C., & Mundt, C. (2008). Was ist eine psychische Störung? In: S. C. Herpertz, F. Caspar, & C. Mundt (Eds.), *Störungsorientierte Psychotherapie* (pp. 3–32). Urban & Fischer.

Caspar, F., Herpertz, S. C., & Lieb, K. (2017a). Was ist eine psychische Störung? In S. Herpertz, F. Caspar, & K. Lieb (Eds.), *Psychotherapie* (pp. 3–26). Elsevier.

Caspar, F., Herpertz, S. C., & Lieb, K. (2017b). Was ist Psychotherapie? In S. Herpertz, F. Caspar, & K. Lieb (Eds.), *Psychotherapie* (pp. 27–46). Elsevier.

Coady, N. F. (1991). The association between client and therapist interpersonal processes and outcomes in psychodynamic psychotherapy. *Research and Social Work Practice, 1*(2), 122–138.

DiClemente, C. C., Prochaska, J. O., Fairhurst, S. K., Velicer, W. F., Velasques, M. M., & Rossi, J. S. (1991). The process of smoking cessation: An analysis of precontemplation, contemplation, and preparation stages of change. *Journal of Consulting and Clinical Psychology, 59,* 295–304.

Elliott, R., Watson, J. C., Goldman, R. N., & Greenberg, L. S. (2008). *Praxishandbuch der emotionsfokussierten Therapie.* CIP-Medien.

Frank, J. D. (1974). Psychotherapy: The restoration of morale. *American Journal of Psychiatry, 131,* 271–274.

Freyberger, H. J. & Caspar, F. (2008). Diagnostik und Psychotherapie. In S. C. Herpertz, F. Caspar, & C. Mundt (Eds.), *Störungsorientierte Psychotherapie* (pp. 55–75). Urban & Fischer.

Greenberg, L. S., & Safran, J. D. (1989). Emotion in psychotherapy. *American Psychologist, 44,* 1929.

Haas, E., Hill, R. D., Lambert, M. J., & Morrell, B. (2002). Do early responders to psychotherapy maintain treatment gains? *Journal of Clinical Psychology, 58,* 1157–1172.

Jenkins, S. J., Fuqua, D. R., & Blum, C. R. (1986). Factors related to duration of counseling in a university counseling center. *Psychological Reports, 58,* 467–472.

Kiesler, D. J. (1966a). Basic methodological issues implicit in psychotherapy process research. *American Journal of Psychotherapy, 20,* 135–155.

Kiesler, D. J. (1966b). Some myths of psychotherapy research and the search for a paradigm. *Psychological Bulletin, 65,* 110–136.

Kiesler, D. J. (1969). A grid model for theory and research in the psychotherapies. In L. D. Eron & R. Callahan (Eds.), *The relationship of theory to practice in psychotherapy.* Aldine Publishing Co.

Michelson, A. A., & Morley, E. W. (1987). On the relative motion of the earth and the luminiferous ether. *American Journal of Science, 34,* 333–345.

Orlinsky, D. E., Grawe, K., & Parks, B. K. (1994). Process and outcome in psychotherapy. In A. E. Bergin & S. L. Garfield (Eds.), *Handbook of psychotherapy and behaviour change* (4th edn., pp. 270–276). Wiley.

Orlinsky, D. E., & Howard, K. I. (1978). The relation of process to outcome in psychotherapy. In S. L. Garfield & A. E. Bergin (Eds.), *Handbook of psychotherapy and behaviour change* (2nd edn., pp. 283–329). Wiley.

Orlinsky, D. E., & Howard, K. I. (1986). Process and outcome in psychotherapy. In A. E. Bergin & S. L. Garfield (Eds.), *Handbook of psychotherapy and behavior change* (1st edn., pp. 311–384). Wiley.

Orlinsky, D. E., Ronnestad, M. L., & Willutzki, U. (2004). Fifty years of psychotherapy process-outcome research: Continuity and change. In M. Lambert (Eds.), *Bergin and Garfield's Handbook of Psychotherapy and Behavior Change* (5th edn., pp. 307–389). Wiley.

Piper, W. E., Azim, F. A., Joyce, S. A., & McCallum, M. (1991). Transference interpretations, therapeutic alliance and outcome in short-term individual psychotherapy. *Archives of General Psychiatry, 48,* 946–953.

Piper, W. E., McCallum, M., & Azim, H. F. A. (1992). *Adaptation to loss through short-term group psychotherapy.* Guilford Press.

Popper, K. R. (1994). *Logik der Forschung.* Mohr Siebeck.

Popper, K. R. (2005). *Logik der Forschung* (11th edn.). Mohr Siebeck.

Sachse, R. (2013). Komplementäre Beziehungsgestaltung: Plananalyse und Klärungsorientierte Psychotherapie. In H. Znoj & T. Berger (Eds.), *Die Kunst und Wissenschaft der Psychotherapie* (pp. 57–80). Huber.

Sachse, R. (2017). *Therapeutische Informationsverarbeitung – Verstehen und Modellbildung im Therapieprozess.* Hogrefe.

Sachse, R. (2022). *Komplexität in der Psychotherapie.* Hogrefe.

Shaw, B. F., Olmsted, M., Dobson, K. S., Sotsky, S. M., Elkin, I., Yamaguchi, J., Vallis, T. M., Lowery, A., Watkins, J. T., & Imber, S. D. (1999). Therapist

competence ratings in relation to clinical outcome in cognitive therapy of depression. *Journal of Consulting and Clinical Psychology, 67,* 837–846.
Truax, C. B., & Mitchell, K. M. (1971). Research on certain therapist interpersonal skills in relation to process and outcome. In A. E. Bergin & S. L. Garfield (Eds.), *Psychotherapy and behavior change* (pp. 299–344). Wiley.

4

Complex Problems

It should be made clear here that clients' mental problems are often highly complex and cannot be reduced to simple patterns. It is argued that psychotherapy, if it wants to do justice to clients, must adapt to such complexity.

Some mental problems are, psychologically speaking, not very complex. For phobias, for example, only a model of classical conditioning is needed, and that is rather simple. This does *not* mean that the disorders are not burdensome or do not require treatment: However, it does mean that the psychotherapeutic measures are often relatively simple.

To say it again clearly: Therapeutically, phobias are highly relevant, they are highly burdensome and must be treated!

Nevertheless, they are theoretically and therapeutically rather "simple" disorders and therefore not comparable to highly complex disorders (cf. Sachse, 2022a).

One should also note here that the principle of "Occam's Razor" by no means implies that theories should be "simple": Theories must be as complex as necessary to describe or explain phenomena.

However, theories should not contain any *unnecessary* complexity: *A theory should therefore be as complex as necessary and as simple as possible.*

Many clients, however, present clearly complex problems, for the understanding of which complex models *with many variables and interactions* are needed. This is clearly the case with clients with "personality disorders"

R. Sachse, *Basic Psychological Insights for Psychotherapy*,
https://doi.org/10.1007/978-3-662-69780-1_4

and can be most impressively demonstrated in this area (cf. Sachse, 2019a, b, 2022b; also: Sachse, 1997, 1999, 2000, 2001, 2002, 2004a, b, 2006b, 2013).

Mental problems become particularly complex when it is necessary to differentiate a disorder into specific "sub-disorders" that all require highly specific interventions and strategies (as with personality disorders; cf. Breil & Sachse, 2016; Kramer & Sachse, 2021; Sachse, 2002, 2006a, b, 2008, 2014a, b, c, 2016a, b, 2018a, b, c, 2019a, 2022b, c; Sachse & Fasbender, 2013; Sachse et al., 2012, 2021; Sachse et al. 2014a, b, c; Sachse & Kiszkenow-Bäker, 2016; Sachse et al., 2015; Sachse & Kramer, 2016, 2019; Sachse & Sachse, 2016a, b, 2017; Sachse et al., 2011; Sachse & Walburg, 2017).

Complexity arises not only because individual problems are highly complex and require specific therapeutic strategies, but also because complex disorders in a person *occur together and interact with each other* (Sachse, 2020; Sachse & Kiskenow-Bäker, 2020a, b, c, d).

Such complex problems can *never* be solved by trial and error (at least not in a manageable time, unless one has time periods available like evolution) and they usually also require complex solutions. And: The solutions must fit exactly to the problems, they must not just "solve" anything, but exactly the problem: This implies that one must have analyzed and understood a problem before one can develop a suitable solution.

And these solutions can usually only be developed through complex (and often relatively lengthy) *psychotherapeutic processes*. For complex problems, one usually also needs *new* solutions, since the old solutions obviously do not (any longer) work.

Therefore, a crucial rule applies to a complex problem: *One must understand a problem in order to be able to solve it effectively.*

Complex problems can be viewed *as complex systems*: To change a system sustainably, one must know how it works, *then* one can deduce which variables need to be influenced how and by what means to modify the system sustainably.

Therefore, the rule here is: *Understand before solving!*

Complex problems (and complex systems) are usually not easy to understand: They require elaborate analyses with elaborate methods, and that requires *time!*

And it requires that one forms a complex model of the system, which can serve as the basis for understanding (cf. Haken, 1995; Haken & Schiepek, 2010; Schiepek, 1991; Schiepek et al., 1992, 1997, 2000).

Here, "understanding" is understood in the sense of language psychology as a complex reconstruction process based on data and on the basis of knowledge: Understanding means forming a valid model of the "system problem"! This creates an "explanation basis" for the problem (cf. Bischof, 2016).

This kind of understanding, according to new epistemological and scientific theoretical concepts, is also the goal of science, and it is the goal of every therapy process!

> So, in psychotherapy, one must start from the realization: *A complex psychological problem that one does not understand cannot be effectively solved!*

Therefore, a therapist should always first form a client model and *then* make specific indication decisions.

So: Do not act specifically based on a diagnosis alone and never without a model. In other words: "Never shoot from the hip!"

With relatively simple problems, one can possibly work out solutions without knowing the problem individually, perhaps *because there is no high individual variance here.* To stick with a metaphor: I can change a tire without knowing what damaged it. And I don't have to analyze a damaged tire to change it: With simply structured problems, a so-called "solution orientation" is quite sensible!

The more complex a problem becomes, the less one can follow such a model!

If I have a complex problem with the electronics, then I should know exactly where the problem lies in order to fix it as effectively as possible. Of course, I can also throw away the car and buy a new one. This is a safe, but not really sensible solution, and it is not applicable to people!

References

Bischof, N. (2016). *Struktur und Bedeutung. Einführung in die Systemtheorie.* Hogrefe.

Breil, J., & Sachse, R. (2016). *Klärungsorientierte Psychotherapie der Borderline-Persönlichkeit.* Hogrefe.

Haken, H. (1995). *Synergetik: Die Lehre vom Zusammenwirken.* Rowohlt.

Haken, H., & Schiepek, G. (2010). *Synergetik in der Psychologie.* Hogrefe.

Kramer, U., & Sachse, R. (2021). Persönlichkeitsstörungen: Theorie und Therapie nach Klärungsorientierter Verhaltenstherapie. *Verhaltenstherapie und Verhaltensmedizin, 42*, 190–205.

Sachse, R. (1997). *Persönlichkeitsstörungen: Psychotherapie dysfunktionaler Interaktionsstile.* Hogrefe.

Sachse, R. (1999). *Persönlichkeitsstörungen. Psychotherapie dysfunktionaler Interaktionsstile* (2nd edn.). Hogrefe.

Sachse, R. (2000). Der Einfluss von Persönlichkeitsstörungen auf den Therapieprozess. In: E. Parfy, H. Rethenbacher, R. Sigmund, R. Schoberger, & C. Butschek (Eds.), *Bindung und Interaktion. Dimensionen der professionellen Beziehungsgestaltung* (pp. 85–111). Facultas.

Sachse, R. (2001). *Psychologische Psychotherapie der Persönlichkeitsstörungen.* Hogrefe.

Sachse, R. (2002). *Histrionische und narzisstische Persönlichkeitsstörungen.* Hogrefe.

Sachse, R. (2004a). *Persönlichkeitsstörungen. Leitfaden für eine Psychologische Psychotherapie.* Hogrefe.

Sachse, R. (2004b). Histrionische und narzisstische Persönlichkeitsstörungen. In R. Merod (Eds.), *Behandlung von Persönlichkeitsstörungen* (pp. 357–404). DGVT-Verlag.

Sachse, R. (2006a). *Persönlichkeitsstörungen verstehen – Zum Umgang mit schwierigen Klienten.* Psychiatrie-Verlag.

Sachse, R. (2006b). *Narzisstische Persönlichkeitsstörungen. Psychotherapie, 11*(2), 241–246.

Sachse, R. (2008). Histrionische und narzisstische Persönlichkeitsstörung. In M. Hermer & B. Röhrle (Eds.), *Handbuch der therapeutischen Beziehung* (Vol. 2, pp. 1105–1125). DGVT-Verlag.

Sachse, R. (2013). *Persönlichkeitsstörungen: Leitfaden für eine psychologische Psychotherapie* (2nd edn.). Hogrefe.

Sachse, R. (2014a). Klärungsorientierte Verhaltenstherapie der dependenten Persönlichkeitsstörung. *Persönlichkeitsstörungen: Theorie und Therapie, 18*(2), 119–128.

Sachse, R. (2014b). Klärungsorientierte Verhaltenstherapie der schizoiden Persönlichkeitsstörung. *Psychotherapie im Dialog, 3*, 56–59.

Sachse, R. (2014c). Klärungsorientierte Verhaltenstherapie des Narzissmus. In S. Sulz & T. Bronisch (Eds.), *Verständnis und Psychotherapie der narzisstischen Persönlichkeitsstörung* (pp. 43–51). CIP-Medien.

Sachse, R. (2016a). Persönlichkeitsstörungen. In T. Schnell (Ed.), *Praxisbuch: Moderne Psychotherapie* (pp. 107–122). Springer.

Sachse, R. (2016b). Klärungsorientierte Verhaltenstherapie der histrionischen Persönlichkeitsstörung. *PTT-Persönlichkeitsstörungen: Theorie und Therapie, Hysterie, 20*(3), 213–222.

Sachse, R. (2018a). *Histrioniker – Mit Dramatik, Manipulation und Egozentrik zum Erfolg* (2nd edn.). Klett-Cotta.

Sachse, R. (2018b). Persönlichkeitsstörungen. In J. Sautermeister & T. Skuban (Eds.), *Handbuch psychiatrisches Grundwissen für die Seelsorge* (pp. 541–559). Herder.

Sachse, R. (2018c). *Persönlichkeitsstörungen verstehen* (10th edn.). Psychiatrie-Verlag.

Sachse, R. (2019a). *Persönlichkeitsstörungen* (3rd edn.). Hogrefe.

Sachse, R. (2019b). *Personality disorders.* Hogrefe.

Sachse, R. (2020). *Komorbiditäten bei Persönlichkeitsstörungen.* Hogrefe.

Sachse, R. (2022a). *Komplexität in der Psychotherapie.* Hogrefe.

Sachse, R. (2022b). *Psychotherapie von Persönlichkeitsstörungen.* Kohlhammer.

Sachse, R. (2022c). *Ressourcen erkennen und fördern bei Persönlichkeitsstörungen.* Hogrefe.

Sachse, R., & Fasbender, J. (2013). Interaktionsschwierigkeiten im Therapieprozess bei Klienten mit narzisstischer und histrionischer Persönlichkeitsstörung. In H. W. Hofert & U. Härter (Eds.), *Schwierige Patienten* (pp. 203–214). Huber.

Sachse, R., Fasbender, J., Breil, J., & Sachse, M. (2012). *Klärungsorientierte Psychotherapie der histrionischen Persönlichkeitsstörung.* Hogrefe.

Sachse, R., Fasbender, J., Breil, J., & Sachse, M. (2021). *Klärungsorientierte Psychotherapie der histrionischen Persönlichkeitsstörung* (2nd edn.). Hogrefe.

Sachse, R., Fasbender, J., & Sachse, M. (2014). *Klärungsorientierte Psychotherapie der selbstunsicheren Persönlichkeitsstörung.* Hogrefe.

Sachse, R., & Kiszkenow-Bäker, S. (2016). Zwanghafte Persönlichkeitsstörung. In T. Schnell (Ed.), *Praxisbuch: Moderne Psychotherapie* (pp. 123–137). Springer.

Sachse, R., & Kiszekenow-Bäker, S. (2020a). *Komorbiditäten bei Persönlichkeitsstörungen.* Hogrefe.

Sachse, R., & Kiszekenow-Bäker, S. (2020b). Das Komorbiditäts-Problem. In R. Sachse & S. Kiszkenow-Bäker (Eds.), *Komorbiditäten bei Persönlichkeitsstörungen* (pp. 38–43). Hogrefe.

Sachse, R., & Kiszekenow-Bäker, S. (2020c). Zur Theorie von Komorbiditäten. In R. Sachse & S. Kiszkenow-Bäker (Eds.), *Komorbiditäten bei Persönlichkeitsstörungen* (pp. 44–51). Hogrefe.

Sachse, R., & Kiszekenow-Bäker, S. (2020d). Komorbiditäten von Persönlichkeitsstörungen mit Achse-I-Störungen. In R. Sachse & S. Kiszkenow-Bäker (Eds.), *Komorbiditäten bei Persönlichkeitsstörungen* (pp. 52–65). Hogrefe.

Sachse, R., Kiszkenow-Bäker, S., & Schirm, S. (2015). *Klärungsorientierte Psychotherapie der zwanghaften Persönlichkeitsstörung.* Hogrefe.

Sachse, R., & Kramer, U. (2016). Die Schema-Borderline-Störung. In: R. Sachse & M. Sachse (Eds.), *Klärungsprozesse in der Praxis II* (pp. 75–104). Pabst.

Sachse, R., & Kramer, U. (2019). Clarification-Oriented psychotherapy of dependent personality disorder. *Journal of Contemporary Psychotherapy, 49*(1), 15–25.

Sachse, R., & Sachse, M. (2016). Zur Klärungsorientierten Psychotherapie der dependenten Persönlichkeitsstörung. In R. Sachse & M. Sachse (Eds.), *Klärungsprozesse in der Praxis II* (pp. 241–251). Pabst.

Sachse, R., & Sachse, M. (2017). *Klärungsorientierte Psychotherapie der schizoiden, passiv-aggressiven und paranoiden Persönlichkeitsstörung*. Hogrefe.

Sachse, R., Sachse, M., & Fasbender, J. (2011). *Klärungsorientierte Psychotherapie der narzisstischen Persönlichkeitsstörung*. Hogrefe.

Sachse, R., & Walburg, M. (2017). Fallverständnis und klärungsorientiertes Vorgehen bei Klienten mit narzisstischen Störungen im forensischen Setting. In N. Saimeh (Hrsg.), *Therapie und Sicherheit im Maßregelvollzug* (pp. 245–256). Medizinisch Wissenschaftliche Verlagsgesellschaft.

Schiepek, G. U. (1991). *Systemtheorie in der Klinischen Psychologie*. Wieweg.

Schiepek, G. U., Fricke, B., & Kaimer, P. (1992). Synergetics of psychotherapy. In W. Tschacher, G. Schiepek, & E. J. Brunner (Eds.), *Self-Organization and Clinical Psychology* (pp. 239–267). Springer.

Schiepek, G., Kowalik, Z. J., Schütz, A., Köhler, M., Richter, K., Strunk, G., Mühlnickel, W., & Elbert, T. (1997). Psychotherapy as a chaotic process I. Coding the client-therapist-interaction by means of sequential plan analysis and the search for chaos: A stationary approach. *Psychotherapy Research, 7*, 173–194.

Schiepek, G., Ludwig-Becker, F., Helde, A., Jagdfeld, F., Petzold, E. R., & Kröger, F. (2000). Synergetik für die Praxis. Therapie als Anregung selbstorganisierender Prozesse. *System Familie, 13 (4)*, 169–177.

5

Psychological Causes of Problems

> It should become clear in this chapter that the psychological processing processes and structures underlying psychological problems are often highly complex, and that the same "surface symptoms" can be traced back to very different processes. From this it is derived that therapists must first create an individual, psychological client model in each case before they make indication decisions.

Different problems and "symptoms" *have different psychological causes:* Different variables and interactions form different "problem systems".

One can view the aspects of a problem, the so-called "symptoms", as the directly observable *surface* of the problem, thus as a "symptom surface".

DSM and ICD, for example, capture such symptom surfaces.

However, it is not yet clear which processes these surfaces are based on. With phobias, there is not much variance here; one can often quite safely conclude from symptoms to processes.

However, this is clearly no longer possible with complex problems.

> *Psychologically, one must assume: The same symptomatology, i.e., the observable "symptom surface", can be caused by different causes* (Caspar et al., 2008)!

This can be seen in the example of "social anxiety": The same anxiety behavior can be caused by

R. Sachse, *Basic Psychological Insights for Psychotherapy*,
https://doi.org/10.1007/978-3-662-69780-1_5

- dysfunctional schemas,
- classical conditioning,
- social competence deficits,
- operant "conditioning processes" such as manipulations, and
- by several or all of these components.

And: Even if two clients should exhibit negative self-schemas, this means that the heterogeneity here also means *that the schemas will then differ (significantly) in detail.* Here too, heterogeneity plays a decisive role again.

But this means:

- *From a diagnosis, one can never be sure of the processes underlying the problem.*
- But one must know these in order to derive valid indication decisions.

The mentioned causes of social anxiety *require completely different therapeutic approaches:* Schemas require clarification and processing, classical conditioning requires stimulus confrontation and social competence deficits require social competence training.

This applies in the same way to other disorders: *"Under the symptom surface" clients show a pronounced heterogeneity!* Thus, two clients with a "histrionic" diagnosis have very different self-, relationship-, norm- and rule-schemas, which a therapist can only know *after* an extensive clarification process; at the time of diagnosis, these variables are usually still unknown (cf. Sachse, 2020a, b).

Apparently, therefore, one cannot derive valid indication decisions from a diagnosis or based on a "symptom surface" (especially with complex problems): One always needs a valid client model!

Even a "disorder-specific approach" is therefore not sufficient: A therapist always needs an individual client model (since phobias are very often comorbid with other disorders, as a therapist, even with phobias, one cannot stop at a diagnosis if one does not want to overlook other, relevant problems (cf. Gouzoulis-Mayfrank et al., 2008; Sachse & Kiskenow-Bäker, 2020a, b, c, d, e)!

Therefore, a therapist must always *first* develop a valid client model in the process, *and then only* can he make specific indication decisions and implement specific interventions.

Based solely on a diagnosis (the symptom surface), however, one cannot make safe indication decisions—at least none that would be psychotherapeutically justifiable.

References

Caspar, F., Herpertz, S. C., & Mundt, C. (2008). Was ist eine psychische Störung? In S. C. Herpertz, F. Caspar, & C. Mundt (Eds.), *Störungsorientierte Psychotherapie* (pp. 3–32). Urban & Fischer.

Gouzoulis-Mayfrank, E., Schweiger, U., & Sipos, V. (2008). Komorbide Störungen. In S. C. Herpertz, F. Caspar, & C. Mundt (Eds.), *Störungsorientierte Psychotherapie* (pp. 657–677). Urban & Fischer.

Sachse, R. (2020a). *Die Psychologie der Selbsttäuschung.* Springer.

Sachse, R. (2020b). *Das Persönlichkeitsstörungs-Rating-System.* Hogrefe.

Sachse, R., & Kiszekenow-Bäker, S. (2020a). *Komorbiditäten bei Persönlichkeitsstörungen.* Hogrefe.

Sachse, R., & Kiszekenow-Bäker, S. (2020b). Das Komorbiditäts-Problem. In R. Sachse & S. Kiszkenow-Bäker (Eds.), *Komorbiditäten bei Persönlichkeitsstörungen* (pp. 38–43). Hogrefe.

Sachse, R., & Kiszekenow-Bäker, S. (2020c). Zur Theorie von Komorbiditäten. In R. Sachse & S. Kiszkenow-Bäker (Eds.), *Komorbiditäten bei Persönlichkeitsstörungen* (pp. 44–51). Hogrefe.

Sachse, R., & Kiszekenow-Bäker, S. (2020d). Komorbiditäten von Persönlichkeitsstörungen mit Achse-I-Störungen. In R. Sachse & S. Kiszkenow-Bäker (Eds.), *Komorbiditäten bei Persönlichkeitsstörungen* (pp. 52–65). Hogrefe.

Sachse, R., & Kiszekenow-Bäker, S. (2020e). Komorbiditäten zwischen Persönlichkeitsstörungen. In R. Sachse & S. Kiszkenow-Bäker (Eds.), *Komorbiditäten bei Persönlichkeitsstörungen* (pp. 66–78). Hogrefe.

6

Complex Systems

Both clients and the psychological problems of clients can be understood as highly complex systems. Based on this perspective, important basic principles for a therapeutic approach can be derived from systems theory.

Clients and also problems of clients are so complex that they can sensibly be understood as *systems*.

A *system* is a complex structure of variables that interact with each other in a highly complex way and thereby generate certain problems, symptoms (observable surfaces), etc. (cf. Haken, 1995; Haken & Schiepek, 2010).

To understand a system, the *designation* of the system (i.e., the diagnosis) is by no means sufficient: One can only understand a system when one has developed a *model about the relevant variables and the relevant interactions. This is therefore a central task of therapists in psychotherapy* (cf. Sachse, 2017, 2020)!

Only when one knows how "the system works," can one (from corresponding knowledge → expertise!) derive which variables need to be therapeutically addressed in what way to achieve desired changes.

The view that clients and problems are complex systems has further implications: Briggs and Peat (1990, p. 270) have worked out some important implications:

R. Sachse, *Basic Psychological Insights for Psychotherapy*,
https://doi.org/10.1007/978-3-662-69780-1_6

- To permanently change a system, its structure must be changed.
- In every system, there are only very few *main intervention points* or leverage points where one can intervene to bring about significant, lasting changes in the overall behavior of the system.
- The more complex a system is, the further apart cause and effect usually are—both in space and in time.
- It does not take many feedback loops for the prediction of system behavior to become difficult.
- Neither the leverage points nor the right way to approach them to achieve a desired result are generally transparent. "Neither the leverage points nor the right way to approach them to achieve a desired result are generally transparent."—Could it possibly say here: "… are generally not immediately obvious."?
- "First worse, then better" is often the result when trying to change a system's leverage point in "the right direction." Any change in planning that immediately leads to better results should therefore always be viewed with suspicion.

From this, some conclusions can be drawn:

- Changing a system makes sense when it is changed permanently or sustainably. Therefore, in the psychotherapy process, the long-term effects are more important than the immediate ones.
- For a problem, one must identify and analyze the *central* psychological variables in order to *precisely* address them psychotherapeutically.
- A "surface" can be created by processes that cannot be directly observed, but only *inferred.*

  And these can be processes that are causally quite far from the surfaces. Therefore, their analysis requires long-term, complex analyses, and one can never say, for example: "The symptom is the neurosis" (if one wants to speak of "neurosis" at all).
- One must analyze not only the relevant variables but also their (complex) interactions.

  For example, in the case of "comorbidities," one must determine exactly how the disorders interact (cf. Sachse, 2020).
- The central psychological variables that need to be addressed are usually not evident: This is another reason why the diagnosis does not provide really relevant information.
- Psychotherapy effects also *usually do not progress linearly,* but often a deterioration occurs before an improvement.

For example, if a client confronts his self-esteem burdening schemas in a therapy process, this often goes hand in hand with a *deterioration* in mood: This is practically unavoidable!

However, when viewing clients and problems as complex systems, these aspects have important implications for psychotherapy:

- Therapeutically, one must *sustainably* change the structure of the system.
- To do this, one must first understand the system.
- One must target the relevant "switch points" of the system: The therapeutic starting points are not arbitrary, but must be precisely specified.
- Finding these central starting points is often necessary, difficult, and requires time.
- However, one cannot *force* this process: It takes as long as it is necessary. Any "hasty analysis" or premature solution approach can quickly lead to errors.
- In complex systems, the central starting points are usually not obvious and not easily observable: Finding them requires systematic analyses.
- It is also difficult to find suitable interventions.
- The effect of interventions must be constantly monitored and reviewed.
- Change processes usually do *not* proceed linearly in the case of complex problems.

A therapeutic approach of the kind "Diagnosis → Indication decision → Planning → Implementation" can apparently only work with very simple disorders, where there is no high interindividual variance, and thus no high heterogeneity.

A priori, i.e., *before* a more detailed analysis, a therapist cannot know how complex a problem really is (e.g., due to the highly probable comorbidities).

If a client has a phobic fear as well as a personality disorder, the therapist cannot treat this if he overlooks it. Thus, he may be able to effectively eliminate the fear *under certain circumstances*, but the actual, significantly more serious problem is *not* treated!

This is neither therapeutically sensible nor ethically justifiable.

Often, phobias and personality disorders interact in such a way that a therapist cannot treat the fear if he overlooks the personality disorder (see Sachse, 2020).

References

Briggs, J., & Peat, F. D. (1990). *Die Entdeckung des Chaos*. Carl Hanser.
Haken, H. (1995). *Synergetik: Die Lehre vom Zusammenwirken*. Rowohlt.
Haken, H., & Schiepek, G. (2010). *Synergetik in der Psychologie*. Hogrefe.
Sachse, R. (2017). *Therapeutische Informationsverarbeitung – Verstehen und Modellbildung im Therapieprozess*. Hogrefe.
Sachse, R. (2020). *Komorbiditäten bei Persönlichkeitsstörungen*. Hogrefe.

7

Therapy Process

It should be made clear here that therapeutic *processes* are of crucial importance at both the client level and the level of therapist-client interaction in the psychotherapy of complex problems. It becomes clear that such processes can never be completely predicted or fully determined by therapeutic interventions. The implications for psychotherapy are discussed.

In the case of complex problems, the solution usually does not come quickly: The problem must first be precisely analyzed and understood, and a *model* must be created. Therapeutic conclusions must be drawn from the model. Therapeutic interventions and strategies must be used to specifically influence the system.

Therefore, psychotherapy presents itself as a complex, lengthy *process* (see Crits-Christoph et al., 2013).

This process must be processed very precisely by the therapist, on a micro level, i.e., a level of individual interventions and individual client actions (see Babl et al., 2020, 2022; Baumann, 1984; Grandjean et al., 2021; Kramer et al., 2015, 2018a, b, 2020; Kramer & Sachse, 2013; Maccaferri et al., 2020; Mailland et al., 2020; Sachse, 1990a, b, c, 1992a, b, 1995, 2003, 2016; Sachse & Sachse, 2009; Sachse & Takens, 2003; Signer et al., 2019).

R. Sachse, *Basic Psychological Insights for Psychotherapy*,
https://doi.org/10.1007/978-3-662-69780-1_7

For the clients, this means:

- They must deal with their own content such as schemas, assumptions, expectations, conflicts, etc. (under the guidance of the therapist).
- For this, they need *trust in the therapist and confidence in themselves.*
- These prerequisites often have to be established by the therapist first.
- Clients then have to *clarify* relevant schemas, motives, etc., i.e., work out a valid cognitive reconstruction of these aspects.
- They must then therapeutically process, dispute, inhibit these aspects, etc.

All of this takes time and can only happen in a relatively elaborate *process: a process that must be carried out by the client and controlled by the therapist.*

This process is also highly complex.

And: *The process of therapy is highly significant in itself, it should be observed very carefully by the therapist and it must also be thoroughly researched* (Lambert, 1992; Lambert & Barley, 2002, 2008; Lambert & Bergin, 1973, 1994; Lambert et al., 1978; Lambert & Ogles, 2016; see Orlinsky & Howard, 1978, 1986; Orlinsky et al., 2004, 1994).

Therapists *continually intervene in the process through interventions* and many variables play a role in shaping the process on the client side.

Theoretically, these processes and *chaos-theoretical aspects* can be considered (see Argyris et al., 2010, 2017; Gleick, 1990; Kriz, 1992; Kriz & Techacher, 2017; Morfill & Scheingraber, 1991; Peitgen et al., 1998; Schiepek et al., 1997, 2000).

Although a therapist tries to control the process, on the client side *many things can happen in unpredictable ways.*

A client can, for example,

- follow the interventions of the therapist,
- intend to follow him, but (for complex reasons) not be able to,
- *avoid,* that is, not follow the intervention, but implement various avoidance strategies,
- suddenly become emotional due to the topics discussed,
- for example, due to therapeutic interventions, fall into a current crisis of trust towards the therapist,
- stumble upon important new topics and thus change the subject, etc. etc.

Even if a therapist can anticipate some of these processes due to his expertise, he can never make a 100 percent prediction about what will happen next in the process.

The process of therapy can therefore never be completely predicted.

A therapist exercises *a significant influence on the client process through his interventions:* If this were not the case, psychotherapy would not be possible at all.

Process research studies (Sachse, 1992a, 2016, 2022; Sachse & Sachse, 2009) have clearly shown *that the influence of the therapist is limited:* A client follows the therapeutic interventions to a maximum of 70 percent—but only under very favorable therapy conditions.

Many variables impair the control effect, sometimes significantly, for example:

- the type of disorder,
- the state of psychotherapy,
- the severity of the disorder,
- lack of trust in the therapist,
- high avoidance,
- unfavorable interventions by the therapist, etc.

Overview

This means: Even if a therapist has some influence on the client process, this influence is *never complete!*

The therapist *steers* the client process to a certain extent, but can *never determine it.*

The process always shows characteristics that can be described *chaotically.*

Despite therapeutic interventions, anything can happen in the client process at any time, much of which a therapist cannot anticipate.

This means:

- A therapist never has the process *completely under control.*
- The process is therefore *not deterministic.*
- The therapist must always expect that unforeseen sub-processes will occur.
- And he must notice this and adjust therapeutically accordingly.

Therefore, a therapist needs not only a client model, i.e., a model of the client's "psychological functioning" and problems.

He always also needs a *process model,* i.e., a model that contains, for example, information about:

- how the *current* trust of the client in the therapist is,
- how strongly the client *currently* avoids,
- how exactly the client *currently* deals with therapeutic interventions,
- what *at the moment* are relevant topics,
- and: which interventions and strategies *at the moment* make sense and which do not.

A therapist should therefore always be *process-oriented* when dealing with complex problems: *The quality of the client process is crucial for the therapeutic outcome!*

It is therefore useful to view the therapy process from a chaos theoretical perspective: An important implication of a chaos theoretical process view is also the realization that processes do not proceed *linearly.*

This can be easily recognized in many courses, e.g.

- the emotional state of clients deteriorates in the process as soon as they reduce their avoidance and face problems,
- therapeutic changes usually do not occur "suddenly", but slowly, step by step,
- clients often take two steps forward and one step back: A client may, for example, have gained a significant insight in one hour and have "forgotten" it in the next hour—apparently, the avoidance in the meantime has "shredded" all insights;
- phases of constructive work alternate with phases of avoidance: This applies to the process as a whole as well as to the process within a therapy session;
- extra-therapeutic events can worsen the client's condition again and thus lead to "relapses" etc. etc.

In view of such considerations, the assumption that psychotherapy processes are linear can only be described as naive.

The essential implications of this are,

- that therapists should intervene as constructively as possible in order to achieve a "maximum" steering effect at all;
- *that therapists must constantly monitor and understand the process,*
- that therapists should be able to intervene quickly and appropriately.

Again, it becomes clear that a therapist should apparently have a high level of expertise.

But if a therapist can only control processes to a certain extent and can never fully predict them, and the prediction (like the weather) becomes increasingly inaccurate the further a forecast extends into the future, a therapist can

- in principle define *process goals*, i.e., those that should be achieved after some time,
- *but never make an exact plan, because a plan can be thwarted by the client at any time.*

However, the assumption that one can plan a process in detail and also over longer periods of time appears completely naive: This is apparently only possible if the process is highly predictable due to low complexity or *if one imposes a process on clients,* i.e., does not respond to what a client does, but puts them in a "straitjacket". Presumably, many clients will not put up with this or the therapist will be treating "past the client".

Therefore, a therapist who carries out an anxiety manual, but overlooks another, complex disorder, can certainly effectively treat the *anxiety*: With this, he can "demonstrate a therapy success"—only: *How relevant is it to the client?*

References

Argyris, J., Faust, G., Haase, M., & Friedrich, R. (2010). *Die Erforschung des Chaos. Eine Einführung in die Theorie nichtlinearer Systeme*. Springer.

Argyris, J., Faust, G., Haase, M., & Friedrich, R. (2017). *Die Erforschung des Chaos. Dynamische Systeme*. Springer Vieweg.

Babl, A., Gomez Penedo, J. M., Berger, T., Schneider, M., Sachse, R., & Kramer, U. (2020). Chance processes in psychotherapy for patients presenting with histrionic personality disorder. Submitted to publication. *Journal of clinical psychology*.

Babl, A., Berger, T., Eubanks, C. F., Gomez Penedo, J., Caspar, F., Sachse, R., & Kramer, U. (2022). Addressing interpersonal patterns in patients with personality disorder explains psychotherapy outcome: A mediation analysis. *Psychotherapy Research, 32*(8), 984–994.

Baumann, U. (1984). *Makro-/Mikroperspektive*. Hogrefe.

Crits-Christoph, P., Connolly Gibbons, M. B., & Mukherjee, D. (2013). Psychotherapy process-outcome research. In M. J. Lambert (Eds.), *Handbook of psychotherapy and behavior change* (pp. 298–339). Wiley.

Gleick, J. (1990). *Chaos – Die Ordnung des Universums*. Droemersche Verlagsanstalt Knaur.

Grandjean, L., Hummel, J., Wyer, D., Beuchat, H., Caspar, F., Sachse, R., Berger, T., & Kramer, U. (2021). Psychotherapeutic case formulation: Plan analysis for narcissistic personality disorder. *Personality and Mental Health, 15*(4), 309–316.

Kramer, U., & Sachse, R. (2013). Early clarification processes in client presenting with borderline personality disorder: Relations with symptom level and change. *Person-centered & Experiential Psychotherapies, 12*(2), 157–175.

Kramer, U., Gholam, M., Maillard, P., Kolly, S., Püschel, O., & Sachse, R. (2020). *Subtypes of narcissistic personality disorder based on psychotherapy process: A longitudinal non-parametric analysis*. In Press.

Kramer, U., Pascual-Leone, A., Rohde, K. B., & Sachse, R. (2015). Emotional processing, interaction process, and outcome in clarification-oriented psychotherapy for personality disorders: A process-outcome analysis. *Journal of Personality Disorders, 29*, 1–19.

Kramer, U., Pascual-Leone, A., Rohde, K. B., & Sachse, R. (2018a). The role of shame and self-compassion in psychotherapy for narcissistic personality disorder: An exploratory study. *Clinical psychology & psychotherapy, 25*(2), 272–282.

Kramer, U., Pascual-Leone, A., Rohde, K. B., & Sachse, R. (2018b). Emotionale Verarbeitung, Interaktionsprozess und Ergebnis in der Klärungsorientierten Psychotherapie von Persönlichkeitsstörungen: Eine Prozess-Outcome-Analyse. In: R. Sachse & M. Sachse (Eds.), *Forschung in der Klärungsorientierten Psychotherapie II* (pp. 145–159). Pabst.

Kriz, J. (1992). *Chaos und Struktur – Systemtheorie* (Vol. 1). Quintessenz.

Kriz, J., & Tschacher, W. (2017). *Synergetik als Ordner*. Pabst Science Publishers.

Lambert, M. J. (1992). Psychotherapy outcome research: Implications for integrative and eclectic therapists. In J. C. Norcross & M. R. Goldfried (Eds.), *Handbook of psychotherapy integration* (pp. 94–129). Basic Books.

Lambert, M. J., & Barley, D. E. (2002). Research summary on the therapeutic relationship and psychotherapy outcome. In J. C. Norcross (Eds.), *Psychotherapy relationships that work* (pp. 17–36). University Press.

Lambert, M. J., & Barley, D. E. (2008). Die therapeutische Beziehung und der Psychotherapieeffekt – Eine Übersicht empirischer Forschungsergebnisse. In M. Hermer & B. Röhrle (Eds.), *Handbuch der therapeutischen Beziehung* (Vol. 1, pp. 109–139). DGVT-Verlag.

Lambert, M. J., & Bergin, A. E. (1973). Psychotherapeutic outcomes and issues related to behavioral and humanistic approaches. *Cornell Journal of Social Relations, 8*, 47–61.

Lambert, M. J., & Bergin, A. E. (1994). The effectiveness of psychotherapy. In A. E. Bergin & S. L. Garfield (Eds.), *Handbook of psychotherapy and behavior change: An empirical analysis* (4th edn., pp. 143–189). Wiley.

Lambert, M. J., DeJulio, S. S., & Stein, D. M. (1978). Therapist interpersonal skills: Process, outcome, methodological considerations and recommendations for future research. *Psychological Bulletin, 85,* 467–489.

Lambert, M. J., & Ogles, B. M. (2016). Treatment Outcome Studies. In J. C. Norcross, G. R. VandenBos, & D. K. Freedheim (Eds.), *APA Handbook of Clinical Psychology* (pp. 465–477). American Psychological Association.

Maccaferri, G.E., Dunker-Scheuner, D., de Roten, Y., Desplant, J.-M., Sachse, R., & Kramer, U. (2020). *Psychotherapy of dependent personality disorder: The relationship of patient-therapist interactions to outcome.* Submitted to publication.

Maillard, O., Berthoud, L., Kolly, S., Sachse, R., & Kramer, U. (2020). Processes of change in psychotherapy for narcissistic personality disorder. *Journal of Personality Disorders, 34,* 63–79.

Morfill, G., & Scheingraber, H. (1991). *Chaos ist überall ... und es funktioniert.* Ullstein.

Orlinsky, D. E., Grawe, K., & Parks, B. K. (1994). Process and outcome in psychotherapy. In A. E. Bergin & S. L. Garfield (Eds.), *Handbook of psychotherapy and behaviour change* (4th edn., pp. 270–276). Wiley.

Orlinsky, D. E., & Howard, K. I. (1978). The relation of process to outcome in psychotherapy. In S. L. Garfield & A. E. Bergin (Eds.), *Handbook of psychotherapy and behaviour change* (2nd edn., pp. 283–329). Wiley.

Orlinsky, D. E., & Howard, K. I. (1986). Process and outcome in psychotherapy. In A. E. Bergin & S. L. Garfield (Eds.), *Handbook of psychotherapy and behavior change* (1st edn., pp. 311–384). Wiley.

Orlinsky, D. E., Ronnestad, M. L., & Willutzki, U. (2004). Fifty years of psychotherapy process-outcome research: Continuity and change. In M. Lambert (Eds.), *Bergin and Garfield's Handbook of Psychotherapy and Behavior Change* (5th edn., pp. 307–389). Wiley.

Peitgen, H. O., Jürgens, H., & Saupe, D. (1998). *Chaos – Bausteine der Ordnung.* Rowohlt.

Sachse, R. (1990a). Acting purposefully in client-centered therapy. In P. J. D. Drenth, J. A. Sergeant, & R.-J. Takens (Eds.), *European perspectives in psychology* (1st edn., pp. 65–80). Wiley.

Sachse, R. (1990b). Concrete interventions are crucial: The influence of therapist's processing-proposals on the client's intra-personal exploration. In G. Lietaer, J. Rombauts, & R. van Balen (Eds.), *Client-centered and experiential psychotherapy in the nineties* (pp. 295–308). University Press.

Sachse, R. (1990c). The influence of therapists' processing proposals on the explication process of the client. *Person-Centered Review, 5,* 321–344.

Sachse, R. (1992a). *Zielorientierte Gesprächspsychotherapie – Eine grundlegende Neukonzeption.* Hogrefe.

Sachse, R. (1992b). Differential effects of processing proposals and content references on the explication process of clients with different starting conditions. *Psychotherapy Research, 4,* 235–251.

Sachse, R. (1995). *Explizierungsprozesse in Heuristischer und Psychoanalytischer Therapie.* Ein Beitrag zum Projekt „Psychotherapeutische Einzelfall-Prozeßforschung (PEP)". Berichte aus der Arbeitseinheit Klinische Psychologie, Fakultät für Psychologie, Ruhr-Universität Bochum.

Sachse, R. (2003). *Klärungsorientierte Psychotherapie.* Hogrefe.

Sachse, R. (2016). Prozess-Studien zur Klärungsorientierten Psychotherapie und daraus abgeleitet therapeutische Konsequenzen. In R. Sachse & M. Sachse (Eds.), *Forschung in der Klärungsorientierten Psychotherapie* (pp. 13–24). Pabst.

Sachse, R. (2022). *Komplexität in der Psychotherapie.* Hogrefe.

Sachse, R., & Sachse, M. (2009). Klärungsorientierte Psychotherapie: Empirische Ergebnisse und Schlussfolgerungen für die Praxis. In R. Sachse, J. Fasbender, J. Breil, & O. Püschel (Eds.), *Grundlagen und Konzepte Klärungsorientierter Psychotherapie* (pp. 232–252). Hogrefe.

Sachse, R., & Takens, R. J. (2003). *Klärungsprozesse in der Psychotherapie.* Hogrefe.

Schiepek, G., Kowalik, Z. J., Schütz, A., Köhler, M., Richter, K., Strunk, G., Mühlnickel, W., & Elbert, T. (1997). Psychotherapy as a chaotic process I. Coding the client-therapist-interaction by means of sequential plan analysis and the search for chaos: A stationary approach. *Psychotherapy Research, 7,* 173–194.

Schiepek, G., Ludwig-Becker, F., Helde, A., Jagdfeld, F., Petzold, E. R., & Kröger, F. (2000). Synergetik für die Praxis. Therapie als Anregung selbstorganisierender Prozesse. *System Familie, 13 (4),* 169–177.

Signer, S., Jansen, R. E., Sachse, R., Caspar, F., & Kramer, U. (2019). Social interaction patterns, therapist responsiveness, and outcome in treatments for borderline personality disorder. *Psychology and psychotherapy: Theory, research and practice,* 1–18.

8

Communication Processes

In the process of therapy, communication between the therapist and client takes a central position. It is important to distinguish between different levels of communication. Verbal, paraverbal, and nonverbal levels of communication should be considered. Such aspects can and should be integrated into a concept of psychotherapy.

Many relevant processes of therapy take place "in" the therapist or "in" the client: They are indeed *accessible,* but not directly observable.

However, there is also an aspect that is (more or less well) observable: *the process of communication between client and therapist.*

The therapist forms models and implements interventions. For these to be effective, he must send the client appropriate *messages, thus expressing his interventions linguistically,* so that the client can understand and implement them.

What affects a client are neither the thoughts nor attitudes of a therapist, but *always only concrete actions.*

The client must *process* the intervention coming from the therapist and then initiates certain internal processes (e.g., clarification, avoidance, etc.).

The client then communicates the result of this process to the therapist.

As with any communication process, there are also three levels of communication in the therapeutic context (cf. Ekman, 1999; Scherer, 1993, 1996):

- the verbal,
- the paraverbal, and

R. Sachse, *Basic Psychological Insights for Psychotherapy*,
https://doi.org/10.1007/978-3-662-69780-1_8

- the nonverbal level.

Verbal means that a speaker explicitly puts what he wants to convey into words and linguistic statements.

It can be assumed that the verbal level is usually the central level of therapeutic communication.

Paraverbal means that the speaker shapes a statement in a certain way, e.g.

- through targeted pauses,
- through elongations,
- through volume,
- through pitch or voice position, etc.

With this, he can pursue various intentions:

- For example, he can emphasize certain aspects by stressing them and thus mark them as particularly relevant.
- He can pronounce certain aspects more quietly, thereby making it clear that they are less relevant, etc.

Nonverbal means that a client provides information about

- facial expressions,
- gestures,
- body posture,
- distance, etc.

Here too, a speaker can emphasize or relativize certain verbal contents through gestures.

It can be assumed,

- that the verbal level is the central communication level of therapy,
- that nonverbal and paraverbal channels also convey relevant information that a therapist should definitely consider,
- that communication at the content or processing level (see below) is primarily verbal (accompanied by nonverbal or paraverbal information),
- that at the relationship level, however, communication is largely nonverbal or paraverbal.

Sympathy is strongly conveyed through voice pitch and tone, eye contact, body orientation, close distance to the interaction partner, etc.

Mistrust is also largely conveyed through these channels:

- through body aversion,
- through crossed arms,
- through corresponding facial expressions,
- through reduced eye contact,
- through a reduction of gestures,
- through so-called "manipulators", i.e., self-touches of the client (e.g., rubbing the ear, scratching the forehead, etc.).

The information that the respective channels convey can be *consistent*: Thus, a client conveys trust to the therapist both verbally and paraverbally.

The different channels can emphasize different content aspects differently, however, they *complement* each other to form a consistent overall picture.

However, the other case is particularly interesting from a therapeutic perspective: that the information transmitted through the three channels *contradicts* each other.

For example,

- a client may explicitly tell the therapist that they feel comfortable, but all nonverbal indicators suggest the opposite (e.g., tense face, tense body posture, etc.);
- a client may verbally signal to the therapist that they trust them, but nonverbal and paraverbal indicators suggest otherwise (e.g., turned away body posture, crossed arms, hesitant speech, etc.).

Such types of contradictions are referred to as *signal incongruities*. These incongruities are an important source of information for the therapist: they signal that something may not be right.

When a therapist perceives such incongruities, they should ask themselves:

- What information does the verbal channel convey?
- What information do the paraverbal and nonverbal channels convey?
- In what respect do the pieces of information contradict each other?
- What causes the contradiction?

- Is it relevant and possible to make the client aware of this contradiction? *Not to reprimand them,* but only to offer them clarification, as contradictions are often very relevant clues in the therapy process.

People *always send* information on all three levels. And interaction partners can perceive and "decode" all these levels.

> However, one thing is certain: *A person always focuses (intentionally) on only one level.*

This is already evident from the fact of a person's limited information processing capacity!

That is, a person

- *sends* consciously only on one channel, i.e., they focus on sending information through this channel;
- however, they also always (automatically) send information on both other channels;
- nevertheless, the *focus* of the message is always only on *one* channel.

The same applies to the *processing* of information on the listener's side: *A listener can also consciously focus on only one channel.* On this channel, the person perceives the information well and can process it well. Although there are always automated (intuitive) processing processes that also process part of the information from other channels—this processing is only rudimentary, and much information will escape the person.

A person can intentionally shift their attention: They then focus on one channel and largely block out the other channels. They can do this on the sending level: They then focus on sending information primarily through this channel.

But they can also do this on the processing level: They then mainly focus on one channel and largely block out the others.

Messages are now transmitted on these three communication channels on three levels (cf. Sachse, 2003):

- on the content level,
- on the processing level, and
- on the relationship level.

The *content level* refers to the aspects *about which* is spoken, i.e., about problems, cognitions, goals, disputations, etc.

The *processing level* is about the question of *how* a client works: whether they engage with the therapist's interventions, avoid them, etc.

The *relationship level* is about signals that indicate the nature and quality of the relationship: trust, sympathy, etc.

And here too, both the sender and the receiver can *always only focus on one level.*

For example, a therapist can mainly focus on the content level. Then they perceive all information on this level well. However, they can easily overlook relationship messages that the client sends!

But they can also focus on the relationship level and then perceive and process corresponding messages.

Communication is an exchange process:

- A sends information to B
- B understands this information
- B sends information to A
- A processes this information, etc.

In this process, the interaction partners can understand each other more or less well, respond to each other or not.

> *From these considerations, it follows that therapeutic communication can always succeed more or less well.*

If a therapist sends and receives on the content level and the client also moves there, then communication succeeds: The therapist understands what the client means, and the client understands what the therapist means (at least he can).

However, it becomes problematic when the therapist and client move on different levels. If a client, for example, primarily sends information on the relationship level, a therapist who is "switched" to the content level is no longer able to understand these messages correctly. The therapist then continues to send information on the content level, but the client hears out the implicit relationship messages and reacts to them. The result of this type of communication is that the therapist and client *talk past each other.*

Such a failure of therapeutic communication occurs relatively frequently, *when* therapists largely consider relationship messages irrelevant and/or when they largely ignore paraverbal and nonverbal messages.

This can easily happen when clients with personality disorders primarily send relationship messages, but the therapist, who is not trained for this, processes them only on the content level. This frustrates the client because he feels misunderstood by the therapist (which is also correct). And it frustrates the therapist that his messages apparently do not "reach" the client. In the long term, this is highly likely to ruin the therapist-client relationship!

For therapy, this means that

- a therapist should keep his information processing *flexible*,
- that he must always focus on one level at a time,
- but he must constantly "switch between levels" to "monitor" them,
- and above all: that he should be able to recognize on which level the client is currently "sending", in order to then adjust to the client,
- to understand the relevant message of the client
- and to communicate in such a way that the client can also understand the therapist.

To be able to do this, however, the therapist must again have specific expertise!

References

Ekman, P. (1999). Basic emotions. In T. Dalgleish & M. Power (Eds.), *Handbook of cognition and emotion* (pp. 45–60). Wiley.

Sachse, R. (2003). *Klärungsorientierte Psychotherapie*. Hogrefe.

Scherer, K. R. (1993). Studying the emotion-antecedent appraisal processes: An expert system approach. *Cognition and Emotion, 7*, 325–352.

Scherer, K. R. (1996). Emotion. In M. Hewstone, W. Stroebe, & G. M. Stephenson (Eds.), *Introduction to social psychology* (pp. 279–315). Blackwell.

9

Therapeutic Information Processing

With complex client problems, the therapist's information processing also becomes complex and poses very high demands. Here, principles of therapeutic information processing are developed (based on psycholinguistic foundations).

A therapist must process the information coming in from the client. He must understand what a client says and what he means. To understand the intended meaning, the therapist must interpret the information in the context of his knowledge, he must draw verifiable conclusions from it. For the conception of such understanding processes, one can mainly use psycholinguistic concepts (cf. Bock, 1990; Herrmann, 1982, 1984, 1985, 1992, 2003, 2005; Hörmann, 1973, 1976a, b, 1977, 1980, 1983a, b; cf. also: Sachse, 1992a, 2017).

From a psycholinguistic perspective, one must assume that:

- a person always means something with what they say,
- that "the intended" consists in the person connecting concepts with each other and thus constructing and communicating a *specific meaning*,
- that this meaning can contain many very individual, idiosyncratic contents, which are not easily understandable by an interaction partner,
- that the respective intended can be very complex
- and that it is always much more complex than what is said,
- that the respective intended depends on the activation and combination of certain concepts

R. Sachse, *Basic Psychological Insights for Psychotherapy*,
https://doi.org/10.1007/978-3-662-69780-1_9

- and that the meaning varies depending on the type and connection of concepts,
- that words and sentences therefore have *also* a general, communicative meaning,
- but that they also mean what the speaker wants them to mean,
- which can greatly vary the respective meaning of a word.

Therefore, even for a word (but even more so for complex statements):

- A word has a "communicative meaning", i.e., what is *usually* meant by it.
- But a word does not have a "fixed meaning".
- Depending on exactly what a speaker means, i.e., which concepts he *currently* connects with it, the meaning changes.
- And: What a word specifically means to the speaker is individually different, and therefore potentially highly idiosyncratic.

Therefore, "understanding" is not a simple process. A therapist cannot "put himself in the client's shoes" and never understand "without preconditions".

> *The therapist must rather interpret the incoming (verbal, paraverbal, and nonverbal) data from the client against the background of his knowledge.*

For this, he uses various *"knowledge bases":* a so-called "world knowledge", knowledge about society, culture, social references, etc., psychological and psychotherapeutic expertise, and, as a special knowledge base, also what he has already understood and reconstructed from the client, the client model.

This processing process is difficult, laborious, and complex and is achieved more quickly and reliably the higher a therapist's expertise is.

From these considerations, consequences now result for therapeutic information processing (cf. Becker & Sachse, 1998; Sachse, 1989, 1992a, b, c, 2006a, b, c, d, 2013).

This makes it very clear and very significant that understanding is a "reconstruction of the intended" (cf. Sachse, 1988, 1993, 1996a, b, 2003, 2011, 2022).

And this, from a psychological perspective, is

- always *hypothetical:* Understanding can be more or less "data-supported" and thus more or less *valid,* but it always remains a hypothesis;
- always just a part of the complex pattern of meaning intended by the client.

A therapist

- can therefore *never be sure* that he truly understands what the client means,
- should therefore test, verify, modify the hypothesis, etc.,
- should, as far as possible, verify it together with the client,
- can therefore only slowly understand the client—over the course of the process,
- always has only preliminary hypotheses at the beginning of therapy,
- which he must continue to understand as hypotheses and which he must validate, elaborate and modify.

A therapist must therefore reconstruct *what the client means:* To do this, the therapist can and must use knowledge as a heuristic.

But he must also be aware that, for example, a theory he uses may not necessarily fit a client or may only partially fit. Thus, a therapist can, for example, derive from the existing data the assumption that a certain theory (e.g., about depression) applies to the client. *Whether* this is actually the case, he always only knows *when he has checked it.*

Without such a precise examination, a theory is always just a hypothesis, thus a *heuristic.*

Heuristic means that the therapist forms a hypothesis based on his knowledge and then tests it: Only then can he (provisionally) assume that his theoretical assumption applies to a client and then really helps him to understand the client.

In any case, it is not psychologically sensible to *apply a theory to a client without testing it,* because that would be like shooting in the dark and hoping to hit a rabbit: The theory *can* be correct, but it *doesn't have to be.*

Therefore, "interpretations" of what the client says based on theories (without testing) are absolutely not sensible, and it is also not surprising that they do not work well therapeutically (see Luborsky & Spence, 1978).

From a language psychology perspective, it must also be assumed that the quality and also the speed of understanding as a therapeutic information processing process depend on

- how good and extensive a therapist's knowledge bases are,
- how good and available these knowledge bases are,
- how quickly a therapist can think, how quickly he can draw conclusions, etc.

Because a therapist's information processing should not only lead to reasonably valid conclusions, it should also be *fast.*

To be therapeutically effective, a therapist should be able to process information "in real time". That is, he should be able to process the information as quickly as the client provides it, preferably even faster. And the therapist should have "multitasking abilities": He should draw conclusions, form hypotheses, enter information into the model, test and modify hypotheses, and he should be able to flexibly switch between content, relationship, and processing level. And again, it becomes clear: A therapist should have a high level of expertise!

All such abilities are needed by a therapist whenever *complex processes are involved in therapy,* in which the client slowly approaches relevant information and in which the client gives the therapist more or less strongly "coded" information.

All of this may not be necessary for simple "fear explorations" of phobic clients, but unfortunately not all problems and processes are that simple.

This also shows that training therapists in language psychological concepts is very sensible and should be part of therapeutic expertise.

References

Becker, K., & Sachse, R. (1998). *Therapeutisches Verstehen: Effektive Strategien der Informationsverarbeitung von Therapeuten.* Hogrefe.

Bock, H. (1990). *Semantische Relativität.* Hogrefe.

Herrmann, T. (1982). *Sprechen und Situation.* Springer.

Herrmann, T. (1984). „Sprachverstehen" und das Verstehen von Sprechern. In J. Engelkamp (Eds.), *Psychologische Aspekte des Verstehens* (pp. 15–30). Springer.

Herrmann, T. (1985). *Allgemeine Sprachpsychologie. Grundlagen und Probleme.* Urban & Schwarzenberg.

Herrmann, T. (1992). Sprechen und Sprachverstehen. In H. Spada (Eds.), *Lehrbuch Allgemeine Psychologie* (2nd edn., pp. 281–322). Huber.

Herrmann, T. (2003). Planung und Regulation der Sprachproduktion. In T. Herrmann & J. Grabowski (Eds.), *Sprachproduktion* (pp. 308–331). Hogrefe.

Herrmann, T. (2005). *Sprache verwenden. Funktionen – Evolution – Prozesse.* Kohlhammer.

Hörmann, H. (1973). Semantische Anomalie, Metapher und Witz, oder Schlafen farblose grüne Ideen wirklich wütend? *Folia Linguistica, 5,* 310–328.

Hörmann, H. (1976a). *Meinen und Verstehen: Grundzüge einer psychologischen Semantik.* Suhrkamp.

Hörmann, H. (1976b). The concept of sense constancy. *Lingua, 39,* 269–280.

Hörmann, H. (1977). *Psychologie der Sprache.* Springer.

Hörmann, H. (1980). Der Vorgang des Verstehens. In W. Kühlwein & A. Raasch (Eds.), *Sprache und Verstehen*, 17–29. Kongreßberichte der 10. Jahrestagung der Gesellschaft für Angewandte Linguistik GAL e. V., Mainz, 1979. Narr.
Hörmann, H. (1983a). *Was tun die Wörter miteinander im Satz? oder: Wieviele sind einige, mehrere und ein paar?* Hogrefe.
Hörmann, H. (1983b). Über einige Aspekte des Begriffs "Verstehen". In: L. Montada & K. Reusser (Eds.), *Kognition und Handeln*. Klett-Cotta.
Luborsky, L., & Spence, D. P. (1978). Quantitative research on psychoanalytic therapy. In S. L. Garfield & A. E. Bergin (Eds.), *Handbook of psychotherapy and behavior change: An empirical analysis* (pp. 331–368). Wiley.
Sachse, R. (1988). Das Konzept des empathischen Verstehens: Versuch einer sprachpsychologischen Klärung und Konsequenzen für das therapeutische Handeln. In GwG (Eds.), *Orientierung an der Person: Diesseits und Jenseits von Psychotherapie* (Vol. 2, pp. 162–174). GwG.
Sachse, R. (1989). Zur allgemeinpsychologischen Fundierung von Klientenzentrierter Therapie: Die Theorien zur „Konzeptgesteuerten Informationsverarbeitung" und ihre Bedeutung für den Verstehensprozeß. In R. Sachse & J. Howe (Eds.), *Zur Zukunft der Klientenzentrierten Psychotherapie* (pp. 76–101). Asanger.
Sachse, R. (1992a). *Zielorientierte Gesprächspsychotherapie – Eine grundlegende Neukonzeption*. Hogrefe.
Sachse, R. (1992b). Psychotherapie als komplexe Aufgabe: Verarbeitungs-, Intentionsbildungs- und Handlungsplanungsprozesse bei Psychotherapeuten. In R. Sachse, G. Lietaer, & W. B. Stiles (Eds.), *Neue Handlungskonzepte der Klientenzentrierten Psychotherapie* (pp. 109–112). Asanger.
Sachse, R. (1992c). Informationsverarbeitungs- und Handlungsplanungsprozesse bei Psychotherapeuten. In L. Montada (Eds.), *Bericht über den 38. Kongress der Deutschen Gesellschaft für Psychologie in Trier* (2nd edn. pp. 942–946). Hogrefe.
Sachse, R. (1993). Empathie. In A. Schorr (Eds.), *Handwörterbuch der Angewandten Psychologie* (pp. 170–173). Deutscher Psychologen-Verlag.
Sachse, R. (1996a). Empathisches Verstehen. In M. Linden & M. Hautzinger (Eds.), *Verhaltenstherapie: Techniken, Einzelverfahren und Behandlungsanleitungen* (pp. 24–30). Springer.
Sachse, R. (1996b). *Praxis der Zielorientierten Gesprächspsychotherapie*. Hogrefe.
Sachse, R. (2003). *Klärungsorientierte Psychotherapie*. Hogrefe.
Sachse, R. (2006a). *Persönlichkeitsstörungen verstehen – Zum Umgang mit schwierigen Klienten*. Psychiatrie-Verlag.
Sachse, R. (2006b). Therapeutische Informationsverarbeitung. In B. Strauß, F. Hohagen, & F. Caspar (Eds.), *Lehrbuch Psychotherapie, Teilband 2* (pp. 1359–1386). Hogrefe.
Sachse, R. (2006c). Valide Information entsteht im Therapieprozess: Zur Bedeutung von Beziehungsgestaltung und Klärung in der Anfangsphase von Psychotherapie. In R. Sachse & P. Schlebusch (Eds.), *Perspektiven Klärungsorientierter Psychotherapie* (pp. 281–293). Pabst.

Sachse, R. (2006d). Indikation von Klientenmodellen: Die Bedeutung von Störungstheorie und Einzelfallanalysen. In R. Sachse & P. Schlebusch (Eds.), *Perspektiven Klärungsorientierter Psychotherapie*, 294–305. Pabst.

Sachse, R. (2011). Empathie. In M. Linden & M. Hautzinger (Eds.), *Verhaltenstherapiemanual* (pp. 121–126). Springer-Verlag.

Sachse, R. (2013). Die Rückkehr des Homogenitätsmythos. *Report Psychologie,* 50–52.

Sachse, R. (2017). Beziehungsgestaltung in der Klärungsorientierten Verhaltenstherapie. In *Verhaltenstherapie und Verhaltensmedizin, 38,* 344–359. Hogrefe.

Sachse, R. (2022). *Psychotherapie von Persönlichkeitsstörungen*. Kohlhammer.

10

Heuristics

In therapeutic information processing, so-called "heuristics" play a crucial role: A therapist should develop hypothetical models, but constantly test, elaborate, modify, etc., thereby developing a verifiable client model.

The fact that clients can be grouped into categories, such as "people with narcissistic personality disorder," means that the clients have certain variables in common and exhibit certain variables.

Such categories and models are always *heuristics* in the therapy process, i.e., they are hypothetical models that are tentatively applied to clients, but must be constantly tested and modified. They help a therapist specifically in processing information and understanding complex relationships.

They alert the therapist, for example, to which other variables and processes are likely to occur, what problems and interaction problems he can expect, and which therapeutic principles he should now follow.

Such heuristics therefore have an important function for therapists: They sensitize the therapist to certain information and questions, prevent a therapist from overlooking relevant information, and allow conclusions to be drawn about previously unclear variables and which therapeutic principles he should now follow (cf. Grawe, 1988, 1995).

R. Sachse, *Basic Psychological Insights for Psychotherapy*,
https://doi.org/10.1007/978-3-662-69780-1_10

Overview

What one should absolutely consider when using such categories is:

- They are always (diagnostic) *hypotheses*, which need to be tested, validated, elaborated, modified.
- Even if they are validated by data, they are never "true", irrefutable or immutable, they remain hypotheses.
- A therapist must always validate with data whether this hypothesis actually applies to the client.
- *A therapist must always be aware that clients, in addition to the common characteristics, have many very individual, idiosyncratic characteristics.*

Clients exhibit highly specific motivational expressions, individual schemas, specific actions, etc.

These idiosyncratic characteristics are very important, and the therapist must always clarify and work them out in detail with a client.

They can never be derived from a diagnostic category. That's why a therapist always needs—besides a diagnosis—a client model, and he always derives concrete interventions from this model!

This means: One must also always consider a "diagnosis" as a heuristic!

This also means that a diagnosis *is always and remains a hypothesis and is never "the truth". A diagnosis can be very well validated, but it always remains a hypothesis.*

Making diagnoses as immutable "characteristics" is therefore nonsensical and unjustifiable!

A "diagnosis" is also always a first, rough orientation, a hypothetical heuristic, which can provide important orientations for the therapist.

But it is never sufficient for therapy!

For example, two clients can both receive the diagnosis "narcissistic personality disorder" due to relevant variables (relationship motives, schemas, manipulative strategies).

Then their schemas resemble each other: Both clients have a double self-schema, one of which describes the client as deficient ("failure schema") and the other as (highly) competent.

But: *What exactly* is in the individual schemas is determined by the idiosyncratic conditions in the biography of these two clients. Therefore, for example, the "failure schema" can contain very different assumptions in both clients: These are then highly client-specific, i.e., idiosyncratic!

And: In order to be able to effectively work on *these* respective schemas, a therapist must know exactly what content *is in the respective schemas.*

This means that in addition to a general diagnosis (as a "frame heuristic"), he always needs to work out a *specific client model* with the client!

Diagnoses are an important step, but always only a first orientation for the therapist: After that, the *detailed work* only begins in the therapy process.

References

Grawe, K. (1988). Heuristische Psychotherapie. Ein schematheoretisch fundierte Konzeption des Psychotherapieprozesses. *Integrative Therapie. Zeitschrift für Verfahren Humanistischer Psychologie und Pädagogik, Sonderdruck, 4,* 309–324.

Grawe, K. (1995). Grundriss einer Allgemeinen Psychotherapie. *Psychotherapeut, 40,* 130–145.

11

Client Model

The formation of a client model or individual case concept is essential in psychotherapy for complex problems. This discusses how a therapist can form such a model, at what point they can receive what kind of relevant information, and how such a model should be structured.

As already stated, a therapist should always create an individual case concept or client model in addition to a diagnosis (see Sachse, 1992, 2003, 2006a, b, 2017).

For various reasons, however, this is difficult and time-consuming:

- In clients with personality disorders, a therapist can expect that clients with high *interactional mistrust* come into therapy. This strongly prevents them from sharing self-esteem burdening aspects with therapists.
  Only when a therapist has built trust through targeted relationship building do clients open up: Only *then* do they define their *real problems* and let the therapist "look into their cards". However, this process of building trust is complex and takes time.
  Based on targeted analysis strategies, a therapist can also draw many conclusions from the client's actions for his model beforehand. But this also takes time.
- Even clients without personality disorders can strongly avoid (e.g., clients with psychosomatic processing structure; see Atrops & Sachse, 1994; Sachse, 1997, 1998, 2006c, 2018a, b): This prevents them from

R. Sachse, *Basic Psychological Insights for Psychotherapy*,
https://doi.org/10.1007/978-3-662-69780-1_11

dealing with relevant problem content. This also prevents the therapist from receiving certain relevant information about the client *not.* Only systematic processing of avoidance gives the therapist access to relevant information.

- Many clients, especially those with high alienation (a "detachment" from their own implicit motives), can only poorly define their problem at the beginning of therapy.
  They often do not even represent all the costs that their system generates (= self-deception), do not know what the important psychological variables are, have false explanatory theories, etc. (see Sachse, 2014, 2020).
  These clients must first work out the costs with the therapist and precisely define what exactly the problem is.

From all these aspects it follows,

- *that therapists are likely to receive only little relevant information from the client at the beginning of therapy,*
- that the therapist can draw conclusions for his model based on certain heuristics, but these are always preliminary and may not reach far. In any case, explicit clarification with the client is necessary;
- that it is naive to assume that as a therapist you already know what the client's problems are at the beginning of therapy and that you understand the problem. As we have seen, diagnoses alone are also of little help;
- that a therapist must prepare for the fact that he must first create the conditions for the client to give him relevant information *in the therapy process,*
- and that this can be difficult and time-consuming under certain circumstances.

This also implies,

- that a client model only *slowly* emerges in the process,
- that a therapist should start building a model immediately, but must assume that the model needs to be elaborated, validated, and possibly modified,
- that client models are always *hypotheses* and never "the truth" and that there can never be absolutely certain models or diagnoses,
- that models can be backed up by *data* to varying degrees, so they are differently valid,
- that client models (and diagnoses!) must almost always be incomplete and preliminary at the beginning of therapy *must.*

A therapist who seriously believes that after conducting an exploration or a Skid interview, they then have a valid diagnosis and a reliable client model, should, in my opinion, burn their certificates. Such an assumption is completely unpsychological and pure wishful thinking. But that's not how clients usually "function".

A model of the client, as can be inferred from the previous analyses, consists of at least two sub-models:

- *The status model* is a model about how the client's problems are currently configured, how the client is currently working psychotherapeutically, etc. The therapist can assume that this model will be accurate for a while: However, since the client (hopefully) changes during the process, the model must be updated repeatedly.
  It is a model about the psychological functioning of the client and the problem and provides a crucial knowledge base for deriving therapeutic approaches, strategies, and interventions.
- *Process model:* As we have seen, the process is partly chaotic and unpredictable: Even a client who fundamentally trusts the therapist can, for example, show increased mistrust due to an unfavorable intervention by the therapist. *Therefore, the therapeutic conditions can change very quickly in the process.* Whether an intervention by a therapist works or not depends significantly on the current *process state* of the client.

Therefore, a client needs, in addition to a (rather static) client model, also a (dynamic) process model: He should always know what the client is doing at the moment and what is favorable and possible right now.

As for the *contents of both client models*, a therapist should make entries on all three therapeutic levels:

- on the content level,
- on the processing level, and
- on the relationship level.

On the *content level*, a therapist should follow guiding questions such as:

- What are the (currently) relevant topics?
- What can be recognized or inferred from the client's problem construction?

- Which psychological processes and variables are important and how do they interact?

On the *processing level*, relevant guiding questions are, for example:

- How does a client deal with the therapist's interventions?
- Does he strive to implement these or does he avoid them?
- Can the reasons for avoidance be identified?

On the *relationship level*, the therapist follows guiding questions such as:

- Does the client trust the therapist?
- How large is the "relationship credit" of the therapist?
- At which points is there also mistrust, and what causes it?

From all considerations, it follows that a client model is the *decisive aspect of psychotherapy*: Without a client model, there can be no meaningful psychotherapy (see Kramer, 2019)!

References

Atrops, A., & Sachse, R. (1994). Vermeiden psychosomatische Klienten die Klärung eigener Motive? Eine empirische Untersuchung mit Hilfe des Focusing. In M. Behr, U. Esser, F. Petermann, R. Sachse, & R. Tausch (Eds.), *Jahrbuch für Personenzentrierte Psychologie und Psychotherapie* (pp. 41–59). GWG-Verlag.

Kramer, U. (2019). Introduction: Case formulation: From the theory to the case. In U. Kramer & M.C. Zanarini (Eds.), *Case formulation for personality disorders*. Academic Press.

Sachse, R. (1992). *Zielorientierte Gesprächspsychotherapie – Eine grundlegende Neukonzeption*. Hogrefe.

Sachse, R. (1997). Clientgerichte Psychotherapie bij psychosomatische stoornissen. *Tijdschrift voor Clientgerichte Psychotherapie, 35*, 5–32.

Sachse, R. (1998). Goal-oriented Client-centered Psychotherapy of Psychosomatic Disorders. In L. Greenberg, J. Watson, & G. Lietaer (Eds.), *Handbook of experiential Psychotherapy* (pp. 295–327). Guilford.

Sachse, R. (2003). *Klärungsorientierte Psychotherapie*. Hogrefe.

Sachse, R. (2006a). *Persönlichkeitsstörungen verstehen – Zum Umgang mit schwierigen Klienten*. Psychiatrie-Verlag.

Sachse, R. (2006b). Therapeutische Informationsverarbeitung. In B. Strauß, F. Hohagen, & F. Caspar (Eds.), *Lehrbuch Psychotherapie* (Teilband 2, pp. 1359–1386). Hogrefe.

Sachse, R. (2006c). *Psychologische Psychotherapie bei chronisch entzündlichen Darmerkrankungen*. Hogrefe.

Sachse, R. (2014). *Manipulation und Selbsttäuschung. Wie gestalte ich mir die Welt so, dass sie mir gefällt: Manipulationen nutzen und abwenden*. Springer.

Sachse, R. (2017). *Therapeutische Informationsverarbeitung – Verstehen und Modellbildung im Therapieprozess*. Hogrefe.

Sachse, R. (2018a). *Klärungsorientierte Psychotherapie psychosomatischer Störungen*. Hogrefe.

Sachse, R. (2018b). Chronisch entzündliche Darmerkrankungen. In: C. W. Kohlmann, C. Salewski & M. A. Wirtz (Eds.), *Psychologie in der Gesundheitsförderung* (p. 639). Hogrefe.

Sachse, R. (2020). *Die Psychologie der Selbsttäuschung*. Springer.

12

Anamnesis

> This chapter critically discusses the importance of taking a medical history in psychotherapy.

Based on the previous explanations, this section will reflect on the purpose of medical histories and medical history collections or "biographical analyses" in psychotherapy.

The purpose of a medical history is to reconstruct the developmental conditions of a disorder and its development over time.

It is highly doubtful from a psychological perspective that this is truly valid (see the studies on the "false memory system" by Loftus and colleagues; Bernstein & Loftus, 2009; Laney & Loftus, 2013; Loftus, 1996; Loftus & Pickrell, 1995), but it will probably succeed in reconstructing certain aspects.

For psychotherapy, the crucial question is how useful or necessary such a reconstruction is.

Many current psychotherapies analyze to a great extent *the current, relevant problem:* They try to create models about the "psychic functioning" of the disorder in order to derive central therapeutic approaches and goals from it. The analysis of current processing processes, schemas, actions and their consequences is in the foreground. Such analyses are, as explained, difficult and time-consuming, but usually provide good models as a basis for effective psychotherapy.

In most cases, then, historical data contributes little to the model.

R. Sachse, *Basic Psychological Insights for Psychotherapy*,
https://doi.org/10.1007/978-3-662-69780-1_12

The basic assumption is that only those psychological variables and processes are therapeutically relevant that actually determine the current problem. Historical data can only contribute to such a model if they can provide new information about such variables and processes and if they contribute to understanding the currently relevant problems. A "collection" of information that does not contribute to the client model is not meaningful.

In some cases, this may well be the case: For example, understanding a client's interaction processes with his father can shed light on the development of certain dysfunctional schemas.

But even in such a case, there is often redundancy: The information obtained from the biography had already been gained from the current analysis.

However, many biographical pieces of information are currently completely irrelevant, for example because they concern areas that have nothing to do with the problems currently being worked on. And then a therapist should realize that he is receiving information *to understand the problem,* not to write a biography about the client.

At the institute, we once had a dispute with an external examiner who described all case reports as completely inadequate because they did not include a "sexual history". Such a statement is complete nonsense from the author's point of view, for several reasons:

- As explained, it is hardly to be expected that a therapist can get many relevant pieces of information about "hot" topics at the beginning of therapy, regardless of the method of collection he uses. Why should a client tell a therapist, whom he does not know, his deepest sexual fantasies and actions? If the client did that, he would indeed be seriously disturbed!
- If it is true that only such information is meaningful that a therapist needs to understand a problem currently being worked on, then information about sexual histories is logically only relevant for sexual problems.
- Otherwise, one would have to assume that *all* problems go back to sexual "basic problems"—however, this is an assumption that is completely untenable from a psychological point of view.

Not only for content-related reasons, but also for economic reasons, the collection of biographical data is a problem: It requires time—and therapy time is extremely precious. Health insurance companies have ensured that time is a very scarce resource. And if you don't want to waste this valuable time, *then as a therapist you have to focus on the relevant problems (you can never solve all problems or "change the client's personality"), and with regard to these relevant problems you have to focus on the data that are really revealing.*

This has consequences for taking a medical history:

- It is apparently very little sense to always take a medical history, and that too in all breadth.
- Rather, one should only collect historical data *when it appears necessary or helpful.*
- And *if* one collects data, one should do so *purposefully:* If one wants to understand, for example, what a certain, relevant client schema is like, one can start the analysis with a targeted question, e.g. through which interactions with which people the schema was formed.

Once you have this information, the medical history is over. Under no circumstances should you let yourself be told "biography" as therapy (in phase 1 of therapy this can be okay if it is used for complementary relationship design; see Sachse, 2016).

And therapists do this for another reason as well: Therapists also only have a very limited processing and storage capacity. And they have to handle this capacity very carefully by only storing *that* which is really relevant, and that too in a well-organized form (see expertise).

> The more information a therapist collects and above all: The more *irrelevant* information he collects, the *worse his client models become,* and the *less* effective his therapy becomes.

Protocols should also only contain relevant information that a therapist can quickly pick up and process again. What use are thick files to a therapist if he never has the time to take note of them again? A "hunter-gatherer mentality" is something a therapist can basically not afford.

> What is crucial is not the "extent" of the information, but its relevance and conciseness.

References

Bernstein, D. M., & Loftus, E. F. (2009). How to tell if a particular memory is true or false. *Perspectives on Psychological Science, 4*(4), 370–374.

Laney, C., & Loftus, E. F. (2013). Recent advances in false memory research. *South African Journal of Psychology, 43*(2), 137–146.

Loftus, E. F. (1996). Memory distortion and false memory creation. *Journal of the American Academy of Psychiatry and the Law Online, 24*(3), 281–295.

Loftus, E. F., & Pickrell, J. E. (1995). The formation of false memories. *Psychiatric annals, 25*(12), 720–725.

Sachse, R. (2016). *Therapeutische Beziehungsgestaltung*. Hogrefe.

13

Psychotherapy and Psychology

This chapter argues why it is necessary to consider psychotherapy as a subfield of psychology, and that psychotherapy should be even more firmly "anchored" in psychology than it has been so far.

Many processes and variables that play a role in psychotherapy are genuinely psychological in nature. Examples include:

- Memory processes,
- Learning processes,
- Motivational processes,
- Emotional processes,
- Communication processes,
- Processes such as reactance, etc., which fall into the field of social psychology.

All these processes play a crucial role in psychotherapy, and they are all part of *psychology*.

What happens in psychotherapy, what goes on in the therapy process, what a therapist influences through interventions, etc.—all of these are genuinely *psychological* processes: *They are the subject of a psychological conception and research.*

R. Sachse, *Basic Psychological Insights for Psychotherapy*,
https://doi.org/10.1007/978-3-662-69780-1_13

One consequence of this realization is that psychotherapy must be considered a *subfield of psychology*, it is therefore neither a subfield of medicine nor of sociology or any other discipline.

From the fact that many and very different psychological processes and variables play a central role in the psychotherapy process, various aspects follow:

- A psychotherapist should *not* only focus on *one* area of psychology, such as learning theory—without a doubt, learning theory is important, but it is not the whole story—; processes of motivation and emotion are also of great importance and may even be more important: e.g., aspects of implicit and explicit motives, alienation, and also the motivation of clients are of great importance (cf. Beckmann, 1997, 2006; Kuhl, 1995, 2000, 2001; Kuhl & Beckmann, 1994; Kuhl & Kaschel, 2004).
  Such eminently psychological aspects cannot reasonably be "blinded out" from a conception of psychotherapy.
- A psychotherapist should have knowledge and a high *expertise in psychology*. This is necessary in order to understand certain processes at all and to be able to derive targeted psychological interventions.

It is unlikely that a psychotherapist who does not have expertise in psychology can practice psychotherapy optimally!

The fact that psychotherapy must be considered part of psychology has further implications: One of them is that one should reflect on which medical concepts are useful in psychotherapy and which are not.

In psychotherapy, "mental disorders" are defined, i.e., unfavorable psychological processing processes and actions. However, these do not have the status of "diseases": "Disease" is a medical term (and a legal concept of health insurance companies), which is meaningless in the field of psychology. (And this applies regardless of what concepts health insurance companies or lawyers demand!)

Good psychotherapy always includes good relationship management. A therapist treats a client respectfully and as a "customer" who has a specific concern.

Therefore, a therapist should never pathologize a client, because this devalues the client.

The term "psychopathology" is not only extremely derogatory, it is also in no way meaningful in psychology: A disorder is a disorder because it causes individual costs, not because it is "psychopathological".

Speaking of "psychopathology" is not only extremely unpsychological, it is also extremely discriminatory!

Psychological psychotherapists should, in my opinion, resist such terminologies!

One can also object to the term "patient": Because "patient" implies that this "patient" contributes little to the diagnosis and therapy, but has to leave most of it to a doctor.

Psychotherapy places *much higher demands on the person:* They must actively participate, actively carry out processes, implement interventions, make an effort, confront content, etc. Therefore, the term "patient" does not fit here, and the participants in psychotherapy are therefore called *clients* here. I do not insist on the word "client", but I think it is a very good alternative to "patient".

References

Beckmann, J. (1997). *Alienation and Conformity.* Max-Planck-Institut für psychologische Forschung.

Beckmann, J. (2006). Konsequenzen der Entfremdung vom Selbst. In R. Sachse & P. Schlebusch (Eds.), *Perspektiven Klärungsorientierter Psychotherapie* (pp. 46–59). Pabst.

Kuhl, J. (1995). *Introjektion, Alienation und Grübeln: Von rationalen Motivationsmodelle zu EEG-Korrelaten volitionaler Hemmung.* Universität Osnabrück.

Kuhl, J. (2000). A functional-design approach to motivation and self-regulation: The dynamics of personality systems interactions. In M. Boekaerts, P. R. Pintrich, & M. Zeidner (Eds.), *Handbook of self-regulation* (pp. 111–169). Academic.

Kuhl, J. (2001). *Motivation und Persönlichkeit: Interaktionen psychischer Systeme.* Hogrefe.

Kuhl, J. & Beckmann, J. (1994). *Volition and Personality: Action versus state orientation.* Huber.

Kuhl, J., & Kaschel, R. (2004). Entfremdung als Krankheitsursache: Selbstregulation von Affekten und integrative Kompetenz. *Psychologische Rundschau, 55*(2), 61–71.

14

Psychotherapy and Philosophy

It is argued that psychotherapy cannot be grounded in philosophical concepts, but that philosophy can fundamentally reflect on and complement psychotherapy.

Having studied philosophy myself, I highly appreciate it. Nevertheless, one should think about the relationship between philosophy and psychotherapy.

Philosophy plays a crucial role in two areas:

1. It serves as an instrument for grounding science, and thus also psychology and psychotherapy: Thus, epistemology and philosophy of science provide important orientations for the development of individual scientific concepts (e.g.: Bauberger, 2016; Ernst, 2016; Hempel, 1965a, b, c, 1967, 1974; Kuhn, 1967; Lakatos, 1970, 1971; Lakatus & Musgrave, 1974; Popper, 2005; Poser, 2001; Stegmüller, 1969; Vollmer, 1975).
   For example, such concepts make it clear that science—despite all its validity—can *never* produce absolute, incontrovertible knowledge, but that our knowledge must always be regarded as a (more or less well-validated) *hypothesis*.
   But it also becomes clear that one should be very careful with the interpretation of "data" and that overgeneralizations can quickly lead to (strong) misconceptions (cf. Sachse, 2022).
2. Philosophy can serve to "transcend" psychotherapy: *Where the individual scientific findings end, a philosophical consideration can begin.* And this

R. Sachse, *Basic Psychological Insights for Psychotherapy*,
https://doi.org/10.1007/978-3-662-69780-1_14

can place psychological and psychotherapeutic findings and concepts in a broader context. For example, conclusions can be drawn about a "human image" and so on.
Such philosophical discussions can all be very interesting, but they are not the subject of an individual science.

One approach is completely unacceptable from my point of view:

Philosophical concepts cannot be used as a substitute for individual scientific concepts.

At points where a psychological theory is needed, one cannot instead apply a philosophical theory and consider that good science. Such an approach was common and even sensible in the Middle Ages, because there were sometimes no individual scientific concepts at all (for example, there was no "physics" and others).

However, the Middle Ages ended in 1492, and since then specific sciences have formed that have developed their own theories. Philosophical assumptions are no longer accepted as a substitute for individual scientific concepts. Sometimes there were misconceptions: For example, Newton still referred to his purely physical work as "natural philosophy" (Newton, 2014), even though it had nothing to do with philosophy.

Unfortunately, there are still cases in the field of psychotherapy where a philosophical theory is used instead of a necessary psychological theory, often without this seeming to be particularly noticeable.

To illustrate, I would like to cite two examples from psychotherapy.

In psychotherapy, the philosophical distinction between "hermeneutic" and "phenomenological understanding" was used. Hermeneutic understanding means understanding based on knowledge and assumptions, whereas phenomenological understanding means understanding a person without any presupposition, i.e., "getting to the person themselves".

From a psycholinguistic point of view, such a distinction is completely nonsensical: *Every* kind of understanding presupposes knowledge, assumptions, etc. Understanding always means being able to classify information in an existing knowledge context (Bransford & McCarroll, 1975).

Something like a "presuppositionless understanding" is not possible at all. One cannot "get to the person themselves" because no one knows or can know what "the person" is. Thus, a "presuppositionless understanding" is a fiction from a psychological point of view, based on wishful thinking.

Another example is the so-called "Focusing" by Gendlin (1969): Focusing is a very good psychotherapeutic method to help a client clarify unclear meanings. The method developed by Gendlin is also effective and we have not been able to improve it (cf. Sachse et al., 1992).

The theory underlying focusing is purely philosophical (which is not surprising, since Gendlin was a philosopher). However, from a psychological perspective, the theory is almost adventurously inadequate because it does not explain psychologically what the goal of focusing is, nor what processes are taking place in detail. We (Sachse, 1995, 2016; Sachse & Atrops, 1989; Sachse & Fasbender, 2010, 2011, 2014) have proposed an alternative theory of affective processing that can psychologically explain why focusing is meaningful and what processes occur during focusing.

If one really takes seriously that psychotherapy is a field of psychology, then one should consistently replace philosophical explanation concepts with psychological concepts.

References

Bauberger, S. (2016). *Wissenschaftstheorie. Grundkurs Philosophie 20.* Kohlhammer.

Bransford, J. D., & McCarrell, N. S. (1975). A sketch of cognitive approach to comprehension: Some thoughts about understanding what it means to comprehend. In W. Weiner & D. S. Palermo (Eds.), *Cognition and the symbolic processes* (pp. 189–229). Erlbaum.

Ernst, G. (2016). *Einführung in die Erkenntnistheorie.* Wissenschaftliche Buchgesellschaft.

Gendlin, E. T. (1969). Focusing. *Psychotherapy: Theory. Research and Practice, 6,* 4–15.

Hempel, C. G. (1965a). The Theoretician's Dilemma. In C. G. Hempel (Eds.), *Aspects of Scientific Explanation* (pp. 173–226). Free Press.

Hempel, C. G. (1965b). The function of general laws in history. In C. G. Hempel (Eds.), *Aspects of Scientific Explanation* (pp. 231–243). Free Press.

Hempel, C. G. (1965c). Aspects of scientific explanation. In C. G. Hempel (Eds.), *Aspects of Scientific Explanation* (pp. 331–496). Free Press.

Hempel, C. G. (1967). The white shoe—No Red Herring. *British Journal fort he Philosophy of Science, 18*(3), 239–240.

Hempel, C. G. (1974). *Philosophie der Naturwissenschaften*. Deutscher Taschenbuch Verlag.

Kuhn, T. S. (1967). *Die Struktur wissenschaftlicher Revolution*. Suhrkamp.

Lakatos, I. (1970). Falsifikation und die Methodologie wissenschaftlicher Forschungsprogramme. In I. Lakatos & A. Musgrave (Eds.), *Kritik und Erkenntnisfortschritt* (pp. 89–189). Vieweg.

Lakatos, I. (1971). Die Geschichte der Wissenschaft und ihre rationalen Rekonstruktionen. In I. Lakatos & A. Musgrave (Eds.), *Kritik und Erkenntnisfortschritt* (pp. 271–311). Vieweg.

Lakatos, I., & Musgrave, A. (1974). *Kritik und Erkenntnisfortschritt*. Vieweg.

Newton, I. (2014). *Mathematische Grundlagen der Naturphilosophie*. Academia Verlag.

Popper, K. R. (2005). *Logik der Forschung* (11th ed.). Mohr Siebeck.

Poser, H. (2001). *Wissenschaftstheorie*. Philipp Reclam jun.

Sachse, R. (1995). *Explizierungsprozesse in Heuristischer und Psychoanalytischer Therapie*. Ein Beitrag zum Projekt "Psychotherapeutische Einzelfall-Prozeßforschung (PEP)". Berichte aus der Arbeitseinheit Klinische Psychologie, Fakultät für Psychologie, Ruhr-Universität Bochum.

Sachse, R. (2016). Prozess-Studien zur Klärungsorientierten Psychotherapie und daraus abgeleitet therapeutische Konsequenzen. In R. Sachse & M. Sachse (Eds.), *Forschung in der Klärungsorientierten Psychotherapie*, (pp. 13–24). Pabst.

Sachse, R. (2022). *Komplexität in der Psychotherapie*. Hogrefe.

Sachse, R. & Atrops, A. (1989). Focusing: Beziehungs- oder Bearbeitungsangebot? In M. Behr, F. Petermann, W. M. Pfeiffer, & C. Seewald (Eds.), *Jahrbuch für Personen-zentrierte Psychologie und Psychotherapie* (Vol. 1, pp. 107–119). Otto Müller.

Sachse, R., & Fasbender, J. (2010). Klärungsprozesse in der Psychotherapie. In W. Lutz (Eds.), *Lehrbuch Psychotherapie* (pp. 377–392). Huber.

Sachse, R., & Fasbender, J. (2011). Focusing: Eine Therapietechnik zur Repräsentation affektiver Schemata. In R. Sachse, J. Fasbender, J. Breil, & M. Sachse (Eds.), *Perspektiven Klärungsorientierter Psychotherapie II* (pp. 131–155). Pabst.

Sachse, R., & Fasbender, J. (2014). Focusing: Die Repräsentation affektiver Bedeutungen. In R. Sachse & T. A. Langens (Eds.), *Emotionen und Affekte in der Psychotherapie* (pp. 156–178). Hogrefe.

Sachse, R., Atrops, A., Wilke, F., & Maus, C. (1992). *Focusing: Ein emotionszentriertes Psychotherapie-Verfahren*. Huber.

Stegmüller, W. (1969). *Metaphysik, Skepsis, Wissenschaft—Wissenschaftliche Erklärung und Begründung*. Springer.

Vollmer, G. (1975). *Evolutionäre Erkenntnistheorie*. S. Hirzel Verlag.

15

Science and Practice: The "Application" of Science in Practice

It is clarified that while a practice of psychotherapy should be based on science, it cannot simply be an "application of science": practice imposes different requirements and pursues different questions, and above all, practice is always far more complex than science can be. The implications of such a realization are discussed.

Scientific research produces relatively valid knowledge. It is the best method for generating valid knowledge that we currently have.

Since research produces such highly valid knowledge, it makes sense to use these findings in practice.

This sounds very plausible, but in detail it is not so simple: *For various reasons, scientific findings cannot simply be transferred one-to-one into practice* (cf. Sachse, 2014, 2022).

In scientific research, the aim is to find as valid answers as possible to questions: One consequence of this is that in research, value must be placed on *creating conditions that can be controlled as well as possible.*

For example, if you want to determine how well a certain form of therapy works for phobic clients, you must

- assemble a sample of phobic clients,
- where the diagnosis of "phobia" is validly made,
- where *all* other disorders (comorbidities) are excluded, as these could uncontrolledly change the results,

R. Sachse, *Basic Psychological Insights for Psychotherapy*,
https://doi.org/10.1007/978-3-662-69780-1_15

- perform a specific, well-defined therapy,
- which all therapists must adhere to,
- try to control or eliminate all "disturbing conditions" (such as the influence of the client's context, etc.),
- ensure that other concerns of the clients are ignored, as they can disturb the "purity of the therapy" and thus affect the interpretation of the results, etc.

These are all necessary conditions for research if you want to get clearly interpretable results.

Overview

However, it also becomes very clear that a scientific investigation creates a certain *context*.

And: *Strictly speaking, these results are always context-related,* i.e., they are also always valid only in a context and validated only in this context.

From an epistemological and scientific theoretical point of view, these results *cannot* be generalized to other contexts (cf. Popper, 2005).

Such a generalization is a so-called "inductive conclusion": And it is by no means compelling and is only possible under certain conditions at all, and even then it is always hypothetical.

You can only generalize from one context to another

- if there are good reasons for it, which can *justify* such a conclusion,
- if there are *no reasons against* such a generalization.

However, it is very clear that the context of practical psychotherapeutic work fundamentally differs from the context of scientific research.

Examples of this are:

- In practice, a therapist must always create a specific client model in addition to a diagnosis (due to the heterogeneity and idiosyncratic processes) and align his therapy with it; this certainly creates a high therapeutic variability.
- A therapist should react flexibly when a client formulates other relevant concerns during the process: Therapeutic goals, interventions, and

strategies can fundamentally change as a result; this is especially *necessary* for clients who only reveal their "actual problems" in the course of the process.

- A therapist who wants to adapt flexibly to the client cannot simply choose a manual and then "beat the client through this manual", even if it becomes clear in the process that completely different client problems are relevant.
- In order to be able to adapt to a client, a therapist must recognize, consider, and respond to the enormous heterogeneity of the client.
- *Thus, in practice, you can never offer the same therapeutic service to two clients.*
- The therapist usually does not deal with a delimited, standalone disorder in clients. Studies show that there is a high degree of comorbidity in phobia clients and that these often require specific therapeutic interventions.

Upon closer analysis, it often becomes clear that a "phobia" is a rather peripheral problem for many clients, which the client "offers" to the therapist at the beginning of therapy because he does not yet want to "put the really stressful topics on the table".

However, it becomes very clear that the practical context is quite different from the context of scientific research: *In the practical context, a therapist is confronted with a much higher complexity, must adapt flexibly to the conditions offered by clients, has little control over such conditions, often cannot consistently implement strategies, etc.*

However, it is clear that the practical context is significantly different from the context of scientific research.

And this implies that one cannot assume that scientific results can simply be "implemented" in practice.

Rather, a practitioner must regard scientific results as important *heuristics*: He should orient himself by them, but he must also check whether they are applicable to a specific client.

Under certain circumstances, he may need to modify, supplement, or perhaps completely discard the heuristic.

Therefore, scientific results can *never* prescribe what a practitioner must or must not do!

They can be important recommendations that a practitioner should know and consider; however, the "practitioner on site" must always decide on their application, not the scientists! Thus, the so-called "gold standard" is a standard for science, but by no means a standard for practice.

There is another reason why scientific results cannot be prescriptions for practice. This is derived from the epistemological insight that science can never deliver "true", definitively valid results (cf. Popper, 2005).

According to Popper (2005), science always produces *"conjectural knowledge,"* which may be considered well-secured at the moment, but which can always be questioned, modified, or relativized by new results and insights.

Even the best-secured therapy studies do not produce "truth", but "the state of knowledge". However, this means that alternative approaches can always be conceived, which can be far more effective than previous ones.

If practice were only oriented towards the current state of scientific knowledge, innovations would hardly be conceivable (and therapy would also in no way be "client-friendly")!

A lively further development of psychotherapy requires practitioners to be able to take new, unconventional paths: However, they should adhere to certain rules and guidelines, such as reflection, supervision, disputation, etc., and they should not consider their own approach as "the true doctrine".

There are also researchers who complain that practitioners do not "implement" research. As explained, implementation is difficult and researchers and practitioners should enter into a dialogue about it. However, researchers cannot make "prescriptions" for practitioners.

Researchers also complain that practitioners do not sufficiently take note of research results: However, the expertise of practitioners is practice, not research. It is nonsensical to expect a practitioner to receive research results in detail. Rather, it would be a task for scientists to communicate research results to practitioners in a relevant form.

It has also been argued elsewhere that the so-called "Scientist-Practitioner Model" is not an ideal solution (cf. Sachse, 2022).

Scientific studies also lead to a self-criticism of science, which shows that even science does not necessarily produce valid results. However, this means that doubts about scientific results may be appropriate.

For example, it is shown that

- the results of psychological studies often cannot be replicated;
- the results of clinical-psychological and psychotherapeutic studies also cannot be replicated;

- follow-up studies of psychotherapy effect studies sometimes yield significantly lower effect sizes than the initial studies;
- studies have errors: errors in methodology, in statistical analyses, and in the interpretation of results;
- sometimes hypotheses are not derived and tested from theories, but post hoc from results;
- studies usually refer to specific contexts (certain disorders, certain clients, certain therapies, etc.)—yet the results are often overgeneralized without apparent justification;
- there are various types of biases: inappropriate results are omitted, "outliers" are ignored, negative results are not published;
- there is also a significant extent of systematic fraud: data are altered, "doctored" or completely invented, etc. (cf. Erdfelder & Ulrich, 2018; Ioanndis et al., 2014; Klein et al., 2014; Yong, 2012).

Science is therefore not "beyond all doubt", the results must be looked at closely, critically questioned, etc. Therefore, scientific results cannot be regarded as "absolutely true" reference points that one can and must orient oneself by.

References

Erdfelder, E., & Ulrich, R. (2018). *Zur Methodologie von Replikationsstudien. Psychologische Rundschau, 69*(1), 3–21.

Ioannidis, J. P. A., Munafo, M. R., Fusar-Poli, P., Nosek, B. A., & David, S. P. (2014). Publication and other reporting biases in cognitive sciences: Detection, prevalence, and prevention. *Trends in Cognitive Sciences, 18*(5), 235–241.

Klein, R. A., Ratliff, K. A., Vianello, M., Adams, R. B., Jr., Bahník, S., Bernstein, M. J., Bocian, K., Brandt, M. J., Brooks, B., Brumbaugh, C. C., Cemalcilar, Z., Chandler, J., Cheong, W., Davis, W. E., Devos, T., Eisner, M., Frankowska, N., Furrow, D., Galliani, E. M., IJzerman, H., John, M.-S., Joy-Gaba, J. A., Kappes, H. B., Krueger, L. E., Kurtz, J., Levitan, C. A., Mallett, R. K., Morris, W. L., Nelson, A. J., Nier, J. A., Packard, G., Pilati, R., Rutchick, A. M., Schmidt, K., Skorinko, J. L., Smith, R., Steiner, T. G., Storbeck, J., Van Swol, L. M., Thompson, D., van 't Veer, A. E., Vaughn, L. A., Vranka, M., Wichman, A. L., Woodzicka, J. A. & Nosek, B. A. (2014). Investigating Variation in Replicability. *Social Psychology, 45*(3), 142–152.

Popper, K. R. (2005). *Logik der Forschung* (11th ed.). Mohr Siebeck.

Sachse, R. (2014). Psychotherapie als Wissenschaft und Anwendungsfeld. *Report Psychologie, 9,* 360–361.
Sachse, R. (2022). *Komplexität in der Psychotherapie.* Hogrefe.
Yong, E. (2012). Replication studies: Bad copy. *Nature, 485,* 298–300.

Part II

Practical Aspects

In this part of the book, practical aspects of psychotherapy are to be discussed, that is, questions about what practical consequences can be derived from the findings.

16

Relationship Building

> The establishment of a relationship by the therapist is an essential variable in the therapy process. Relationship building only has a weak *direct* effect on the success of therapy, but it is a crucial prerequisite for relevant processes to take place at all.

Undoubtedly, a therapist enters into a relationship with a client in psychotherapy. And the therapist can professionally and actively shape this relationship according to therapeutic rules.

He has many options for active relationship building: The therapist can, for example, be accepting, empathetic, respectful, etc. Or he can realize a *complementary relationship building*, for example by forming a hypothesis about the client's central relationship motive and systematically trying to "feed" this motive (see Caspar, 1984, 1986, 1989, 1995, 1996, 1997, 2007a, b, 2008a, b, 2009, 2013, 2019; Caspar & Belz, 2012, 2017a, b; Fasbender & Sachse, 2021; Grawe, 1982, 1986, 1992; Grawe & Caspar, 1984; Sachse, 1987, 1992, 2000, 2003, 2006, 2013, 2016, 2017, 2022).

From a therapeutic perspective, it must be made clear that *relationship building is not an end in itself.* As a therapist, you do not realize it because "you are a good person" or similar. You realize it for very good psychological reasons: *Relationship building creates trust, and the therapist thereby builds personal and competence trust with the client.*

R. Sachse, *Basic Psychological Insights for Psychotherapy*,
https://doi.org/10.1007/978-3-662-69780-1_16

Thus, active relationship building is already a *central psychotherapeutic strategy.*

Such a strategy is, for example, crucial for clients with personality disorders who bring a high degree of interactional mistrust, because without such trust they do not open up, do not give the therapist any relevant information, are not cooperative, etc. (see Sachse, 2019).

Generally, averaged over all clients and therapies, the *immediate* influence of relationship building on the success of therapy is rather low: It explains about 9% of the variance of success data. From this, one could draw the (completely wrong) conclusion that relationship building is therapeutically unimportant. This is not the case in any way.

One reason for this is that in many psychotherapies it is *not assumed that relationship building directly affects the outcome,* but rather that it *affects certain process aspects:* It *enables* further therapeutic interventions and *these* then correlate relatively highly with the success of therapy.

As already stated, through relationship building, for example, one wants to build trust and this results in,

- the client reducing his interactional mistrust and building trust with the therapist,
- which makes the client willing to open up and give the therapist the really relevant, self-esteem burdening information,
- which gives the client confidence in himself,
- can turn to increasingly relevant aspects,
- and is motivated to engage in the process and implement therapeutic interventions,
- which allows a therapist to initiate constructive therapy processes, such as the clarification and processing of schemas.

A *direct* connection between relationship building and therapy success is therefore not postulated. Nevertheless, relationship building is crucial for certain processes to take place at all *can:* How well this works, however, depends again on other factors. Thus, relationship building remains an extremely essential factor for psychotherapy.

Another important aspect is that relationship building is not of equal importance for all clients with all disorders. As Franz Caspar (2008a) says, there are obviously clients who are "relationally undemanding". This includes clients with pure phobias (if [!] they do not have a comorbid personality disorder). These clients show very little interactional mistrust, and the therapist can quickly build trust in competence through good, fast therapeutic measures.

The situation is completely different (as explained) for clients with personality disorders: Without targeted relationship building, therapy practically does not work there (cf. Sachse, 2019).

Considering these aspects, it becomes clear again that averaging the results across clients and disorders corresponds to the homogeneity myth: *You cannot lump together different clients with different disorders.* If you do, nonsense is likely to result!

For example, our process research has shown (cf. Sachse & Kramer, 2023) that for clients with personality disorders, a significant *direct* effect of relationship building on therapy success can be demonstrated.

The *implications for a therapy concept,* that result from this, are as follows:

- Relationship building is obviously not sufficient as a therapeutic measure for most clients. Therefore, psychotherapy cannot be defined solely as a "relationship offer". Psychotherapy must contain much more than that.
- Active, professional relationship building by the therapist is not essential for all clients or all disorders.
- However, there are many clients for whom constructive relationship building is of very great therapeutic importance.
- These clients need a relationship building that exactly "fits" them: The therapist must therefore analyze what a client needs and must implement a highly *differential relationship building.*
- Relationship building, if it wants to be professional, is difficult and requires high expertise from the therapist. The therapist needs knowledge about which clients need what kind of relationship building, and he must implement this well and be able to adapt well to clients.
- The therapeutic purpose of relationship building is only secondary to achieve immediate therapy successes. The purpose is rather to enable further, constructive therapy processes. This results in specific process goals with relationship building that a therapist should pursue.

References

Caspar, F. (1984). *Analyse interaktioneller Pläne.* Universität Bern. Unveröffentlichte Dissertation.

Caspar, F. (1986). Die Plananalyse als Konzept und Methode. *Verhaltensmodifikation, 4*, 235–256.

Caspar, F. (1989). *Beziehungen und Probleme verstehen. Eine Einführung in die psychotherapeutische Plananalyse.* Huber.

Caspar, F. (1995). *Plan Analysis. Toward optimizing therapy.* Hogrefe Huber.

Caspar, F. (1996). *Beziehungen und Probleme verstehen. Eine Einführung in die psychotherapeutische Plananalyse. Zweite* (überarbeitete). Huber.

Caspar, F. (1997). Plan analysis. In T. Eells (Eds.), *Handbook of psychotherapeutic case formulations* (pp. 260–288). Guilford Press.

Caspar, F. (2007a). Plananalyse. In B. Röhrle, P. Schlottke, & F. Caspar (Eds.), *Lehrbuch der klinisch-psychologischen Diagnostik* (pp. 149–166). Kohlhammer.

Caspar, F. (2007b). *Beziehungen und Probleme verstehen. Eine Einführung in die psychotherapeutische Plananalyse* (3rd ed.). Huber.

Caspar, F. (2008a). Motivorientierte Beziehungsgestaltung – Konzept, Voraussetzungen bei den Patienten und Auswirkungen auf Prozess und Ergebnisse. In M. Hermer & B. Röhrle (Eds.), *Handbuch der therapeutischen Beziehung* (Vol. 1, pp. 527–558). DGVT.

Caspar, F. (2008b). Plananalyse. In B. Röhrle, F. Caspar, & P. Schlottke (Eds.), *Lehrbuch der klinisch-psychologischen Diagnostik* (pp. 149–166). Kohlhammer.

Caspar, F. (2009). Plan analysis in action. *Pragmatic Case Studies in Psychotherapy, 5*(2), 25–27.

Caspar, F. (2013). Beziehungsgestaltung. In M. Belz, F. Caspar, & E. Schramm (Eds.), *Therapieren mit CBASP* (pp. 233–250). Elsevier.

Caspar, F. (2019). Plan Analysis and the Motive-Oriented Therapeutic Relationship. In U. Kramer (Eds.), *Case formulation for personality disorders: Tailoring Psychotherapy tot he Individual Client* (pp. 265–288). Elsevier.

Caspar, F., & Belz, M. (2012). Motivorientierte Beziehungsgestaltung. In P. Zobrist (Eds.), *Soziale Arbeit mit Pflichtklientinnen und Pflichtklienten. Theoretische Positionen – methodische Beiträge – neue Perspektiven* (pp. 64–67). Hochschule Luzern, Soziale Arbeit.

Caspar, F., & Belz, M. (2017a). Motivorientierte Beziehungsgestaltung. In E. L. Brakemeier & F. Jacobi (Eds.), *Verhaltenstherapie in der Praxis* (pp. 54–65). Beltz.

Caspar, F., & Belz, M. (2017b). Plananalyse. In E. L. Brakemeier & F. Jacobi (Eds.), *Verhaltenstherapie in der Praxis* (pp. 165–179). Beltz.

Fasbender, J., & Sachse, R. (2021). Beziehungsgestaltung in der Klärungsorientierten Verhaltenstherapie. *Verhaltenstherapie und Verhaltensmedizin, 42*, 162–176.

Grawe, K. (1982). *Implikationen und Anwendungsmöglichkeiten der Vertikalen Verhaltensanalyse für die Sichtweise und Behandlung psychischer Störungen.* Universität Bern. Forschungsberichte aus dem Psychologischen Institut, 1/86.
Grawe, K. (1986). *Schema-Theorie und heuristische Psychotherapie. Forschungsbericht aus dem Psychologischen Institut.* Universität Bern.
Grawe, K. (1992). Komplementäre Beziehungsgestaltung als Mittel zur Herstellung einer guten Therapiebeziehung. In J. Margraf & J. Brengelmann (Eds.), *Die Therapeut-Patient-Beziehung in der Verhaltenstherapie* (pp. 215–244). Gerhard Röttger.
Grawe, K. & Caspar, F. M. (1984). Die Plananalyse als Konzept und Instrument für die Psychotherapieforschung. In U. Baumann (Eds.), *Psychotherapieforschung. Makro- und Mikroperspektive,* (pp. 177–197). Hogrefe.
Sachse, R. (1987). Funktion und Gestaltung der therapeutischen Beziehung in der Klienten-zentrierten Psychotherapie bei interaktionellen Zielen und Interaktionsproblemen des Klienten. *Zeitschrift für Klinische Psychologie, Psychopathologie und Psychotherapie, 35,* 219–230.
Sachse, R. (1992). *Zielorientierte Gesprächspsychotherapie – Eine grundlegende Neukonzeption.* Hogrefe.
Sachse, R. (2000). Perspektiven der therapeutischen Beziehungsgestaltung. In: M. Hermer (Eds.), *Psychotherapeutische Perspektiven am Beginn des 21. Jahrhunderts,* (pp. 157–176). DGVT.
Sachse, R. (2003). *Klärungsorientierte Psychotherapie.* Hogrefe.
Sachse, R. (2006). *Therapeutische Beziehungsgestaltung.* Hogrefe.
Sachse, R. (2013). Komplementäre Beziehungsgestaltung: Plananalyse und Klärungsorientierte Psychotherapie. In H. Znoj, T., & Berger (Eds.), *Die Kunst und Wissenschaft der Psychotherapie* (pp. 57–80). Huber.
Sachse, R. (2016). *Therapeutische Beziehungsgestaltung.* Hogrefe.
Sachse, R. (2017). Beziehungsgestaltung in der Klärungsorientierten Verhaltenstherapie. In *Verhaltenstherapie und Verhaltensmedizin, 38,* 344–359. Hogrefe.
Sachse, R. (2019). *Persönlichkeitsstörungen* (3rd ed.). Hogrefe.
Sachse, R. (2022). *Komplexität in der Psychotherapie.* Hogrefe.
Sachse, R. & Kramer, U. (2023). *Klärungsorientierte Psychotherapie von Persönlichkeitsstörungen.* Göttingen: Hogrefe.

17

Control and Processing Offers

Strong control of the client process by the therapist is indispensable for a constructive therapy outcome. This is shown by all relevant studies. Constructive control is difficult and sensible approaches are discussed.

Process analysis studies clearly show that clients on their own realize only a few constructive client processes. After considering why a client is a client, this is not to be expected.

Therefore, a therapist must *constructively control* the client process and he has, as we have seen, a (more or less strong) influence on the process. He must use this influence (due to his expertise) as well and as constructively as possible.

This means: A therapist must take *process responsibility*.

A so-called "nondirective therapy" has never existed according to all process analyses and is not even conceivable: A therapy in which a therapist does not constructively control client processes is pointless (cf. already Truax, 1966)!

Since clients exhibit many avoidances, unfavorable strategies, etc., a therapist cannot simply offer "developmental conditions" to the client or "leave him space" etc. Because obviously a client cannot use such conditions at all: He rather needs targeted assistance from the therapist.

R. Sachse, *Basic Psychological Insights for Psychotherapy*,
https://doi.org/10.1007/978-3-662-69780-1_17

The therapist always controls through *interventions,* i.e., through specific actions with which the therapist wants to achieve something; interventions that a client must understand and implement in order to achieve the intended process effects.

After everything that has been discussed so far, a therapist cannot, however, regard his interventions as "prescriptions".

Ultimately, it is always the client who decides whether or not to implement a therapist's intervention.

And sometimes he just doesn't.

Therefore, from a therapeutic point of view, it makes sense to consider interventions as *"processing offers"*: They are suggestions to the client to now carry out certain processes, to follow certain questions, etc., because the therapist considers this sensible based on his expertise.

And that's what a therapist should do—he must *control.*

Whether the client *currently allows himself to be controlled,* is another question: The client does not have to and often does not. Therefore, interventions should be considered as *offers.*

A *processing offer* is thus an intervention,

- that a therapist derives from his client model and his process model,
- for which he therefore has good, well-founded reasons,
- and which, if the client were to implement it, would probably influence the process favorably,
- which a client can, however, reject or ignore,
- which he also has a right to do.

Making a processing offer also implies,

- that the therapist never puts the client under pressure,
- that his interventions are "contradiction enabling",
- that the therapist always shows interest in the client.

If a client does not accept the processing offers of a therapist, the therapist can deal with it constructively: He can build more trust, work on avoidance, clarify motivation with the client, etc. If a client still does not accept the processing offer, the therapist may then have nothing more "in the therapeutic offer". But that is ultimately the responsibility of the client.

All considerations also show that the assumption that a therapist has "power" over a client is usually incorrect: The client can easily resist influence, he can decide not to change, he can ignore the therapist's interventions, etc.

The entire therapy is thus an "offer" and not "brainwashing".

References

Truax, C. B. (1966). Reinforcement and non-reinforcement in Rogerian psychotherapy. *Journal of Abnormal Psychology, 71,* 1–9.

18

Interventions

A therapist always controls a process through specific therapeutic actions, so-called "interventions". Important therapeutic principles must be observed when implementing such interventions, which are presented here.

A therapist implements *interventions* in the process and controls the process through interventions (cf. Sachse, 1989, 1990, 1991, 1992a, b, 2003).

Interventions are linguistic actions (accompanied by paraverbal and nonverbal signals) with which the therapist tries to *initiate certain processes in the client.* The processing offers that a therapist wants to make to the client must always be converted into concrete interventions.

A therapist "intervenes" therefore "not just like that": He derives certain therapeutic *intentions* from his model and then implements them into specific interventions.

In doing so, a therapist can pursue very different *intentions*:

- He can draw the client's attention to certain aspects.
- He may want a client to internalize his perspective.
- He can encourage the client to follow certain lines of questioning.
- He can confront the client.
- He can ask the client to dispute certain contents, etc. etc.

R. Sachse, *Basic Psychological Insights for Psychotherapy*,
https://doi.org/10.1007/978-3-662-69780-1_18

As we have seen, the interventions should always specifically control the client process: The therapist should therefore derive from his client model and from his process model which processes should sensibly be stimulated in the client: *This is how the therapist defines process goals.*

And the therapist must decide which type of interventions make sense to achieve these process goals.

Interventions are therefore not an end in themselves.

Interventions

- Interventions always go back to an *intention* of the therapist, the therapist wants to achieve something specific with the client;
- for this, he realizes a certain linguistic statement;
- he must always check afterwards whether he has actually achieved the processes he intended in the client;
- he should plan and implement further interventions based on the result of this analysis.

Here we will now go into a little more detail on the question of how the therapist's interventions should be designed. Process research has shown that therapists can design interventions in such a way that they are highly likely to achieve the desired process goals, i.e. that they have a strong constructive control effect.

Unfortunately, therapists can also design interventions in such a way that they only have a weak effect or even disrupt and destructively influence the client process (cf. Sachse, 1992a).

From psychological findings and results of process research, some *basic principles of intervention design* can be derived.

A psychological result from which principles can be derived that are also empirically well confirmed is the fact that clients have a *limited processing capacity*, i.e. they only have a limited amount of cognitive resources that they can use for certain cognitive tasks. And this also implies: If a client uses the resources for task X, they are no longer available for task Y.

Therefore, a therapist must always implement interventions in such a way that the client can understand and implement them with as little capacity as possible, so that enough resources are still available for other therapeutic tasks.

It is empirically and theoretically unquestionable that many processes that "take place" in the client and should take place are so highly complex that the client can only carry them out *if he concentrates most of his resources on them.* However, this leaves him with relatively few resources for other tasks. This applies, for example, to all processes of schema clarification and schema processing.

If a client, for example, pursues a clarification process, he needs as many resources as possible for this. If the therapist then gives the client another task, the client must withdraw resources from the clarification process, which worsens it (considerably).

Despite all the clarification and processing processes that a client carries out, he must always still provide enough resources for communication with the therapist.

He needs resources to understand and process the therapist's interventions; he needs resources to formulate his statements to the therapist.

> *From these considerations, it follows inevitably that the therapist's interventions must be designed in such a way that the client can process them with minimal resources!*

This results in some therapeutic principles for designing interventions, all of which are empirically supported by process studies:

- *The therapist's intervention should be as short as possible: Good interventions are those that are no longer than 6 words. These have the highest steering effect.*
  Of course, a therapist sometimes has to implement longer interventions. However, he should be aware that he is then causing the client to divert resources from other processes. This is unavoidable in therapy. Nevertheless, a therapist should keep his intervention as short as possible!
- The therapist's intervention must be easy for the client to understand and implement. This implies, for example,
  - that a therapist always *explicitly* makes clear what the client should do: no "messages through the flower", no euphemisms, etc.;
  - that the therapist uses grammatically simple sentences ("psychotherapy is not a German lesson");
  - that the therapist avoids foreign words and technical terms as much as possible!

A therapist should always consider that a client often needs *time to process interventions:* If a therapist wants his interventions to work, he must give the client this time.

This means, for example,

- that a therapist speaks *slowly;*
- that a therapist takes *breaks:* If he has said something important, he should definitely take a break so that his intervention can "take effect".

Otherwise, a client is busy processing what the therapist has said, while the therapist "chatters into the process", thus disturbing the processing.

So: Speak rather slowly, take breaks, always give the client time.

It follows that: The faster a therapist speaks, the fewer breaks he takes, the more information "rains down" on the client, the *lower* the "impact" of his intervention!

This is clear both from the psychological theory and empirically!

All client processes need time—and a therapist must definitely give this time to the client so that the processes can proceed constructively.

The therapist should also *emphasize* particularly important aspects of his message to the client in order to draw the client's attention to exactly these aspects. So a therapist should, for example,

- take a short break before important content: This marks the following content as particularly relevant;
- he should emphasize important content particularly;
- he should also mark certain content as relevant through facial expressions and gestures.

All this helps the client to *focus on the central aspects* and to process these primarily.

Every control that the therapist directs at the client (e.g. "pay attention to X", "follow this question", etc.) must first be executed by the client, and this often requires many resources (cf. Sachse, 1992a).

From this follows the principle: *The therapist should give the client only one task with each intervention!*

If he wants the client to do several things, then the therapist distributes these over *several interventions.*

The therapist gives task A through intervention X; then he waits until the client has carried it out. *Only then* does he give task B in the next intervention, etc.

The *principle of fit,* which will be discussed in the following chapter, also plays a very important role in psychotherapy: Interventions must therefore fit the conditions that a client *currently* has.

This means, for example:

- If a client is in a clarification process at the "level of understanding A", then he should still carry out B and C. This can take time and may require steering from the therapist. But this means that the therapist should next stimulate B and *only then* C.
  If a therapist immediately steers C, the intervention does not fit the client's level of understanding, and the client can at best not carry out the intervention, at worst the intervention also disturbs the client process.
- An intervention should also be adapted to the intellectual level and the level of knowledge of the client: An intervention should not overwhelm the client.

References

Sachse, R. (1989). Zur allgemeinpsychologischen Fundierung von Klientenzentrierter Therapie: Die Theorien zur „Konzeptgesteuerten Informationsverarbeitung“ und ihre Bedeutung für den Verstehensprozeß. In R. Sachse & J. Howe (Eds.), *Zur Zukunft der Klientenzentrierten Psychotherapie* (pp. 76–101). Asanger.

Sachse, R. (1990). Concrete interventions are crucial: The influence of therapist's processing-proposals on the client's intra-personal exploration. In G. Lietaer, J. Rombauts, & R. van Balen (Eds.), *Client-centered and experiential psychotherapy in the nineties* (pp. 295–308). University Press.

Sachse, R. (1991). Spezifische Wirkfaktoren in der Klientenzentrierten Psychotherapie: Zur Bedeutung von Bearbeitungsangeboten und Inhaltsbezügen. *Verhaltenstherapie und psychosoziale Praxis, 23,* 157–171.

Sachse, R. (1992a). *Zielorientierte Gesprächspsychotherapie—Eine grundlegende Neukonzeption*. Hogrefe.

Sachse, R. (1992b). Zielorientiertes Handeln in der Gesprächspsychotherapie: Zum tatsächlichen und notwendigen Einfluß von Therapeuten auf die Explizierungsprozesse bei Klienten. *Zeitschrift für Klinische Psychologie, 21*, 286–301.

Sachse, R. (2003). *Klärungsorientierte Psychotherapie*. Hogrefe.

19

Fit

Therapeutic strategies and interventions only have a constructive effect in the process if they are precisely tailored to the psychological aspects of the client's problems and to the client *themselves.* Such a fit should be established by the therapist.

Considering the enormous heterogeneity of clients, therapists, and therapies, one must psychologically assume that not all therapies or all therapists can be suitable for a client to achieve constructive effects.

Different clients require different types of relationship design, need varying degrees of support, react very differently to directivity, may also react "allergically" to certain therapists, etc.

If one wants to achieve optimal results, it is undoubtedly sensible to offer clients *the* method that fits their disorder, that they can accept, that motivates them to cooperate—and not a method that helps them little or that they do not want, etc. And it makes sense for clients to choose therapists with whom they can build a high level of personal and competence trust, and not therapists who "get on their nerves".

Heckhausen (1969) has referred to such an approach in educational psychology as the *"principle of fit"*, but it undoubtedly also plays a significant role in psychotherapy. *Fit* here means that the interventions, process goals, etc., that a therapist realizes, fit the client, "pick them up where they currently are", and

R. Sachse, *Basic Psychological Insights for Psychotherapy*,
https://doi.org/10.1007/978-3-662-69780-1_19

that they are designed in such a way that a client can understand, accept, and implement them.

The consequences for therapy are clear:

- *One cannot offer the same relationship, interventions, strategies, etc. to all clients.* Instead, a therapist should analyze what a client needs and accepts and, if possible, offer the client exactly what fits.
- This clearly means that not all forms of therapy or methods are suitable for all clients: There is no "one-size-fits-all psychotherapy".
- Since clients are not only seen from their disorders, but are also highly heterogeneous in terms of their personality traits, it may be that therapy X is generally indicated for the disorder, but the client cannot cope with it. *And that's why therapies should not only be "disorder-specific", but also "client-specific".*
- This also means that the therapeutic offer cannot be reduced to two or three forms of therapy, not even because they show "high effect sizes". Instead, a heterogeneity of therapeutic offers should definitely be maintained.

This also makes it clear that *"client-centeredness"* is an important therapeutic principle. Client-centeredness is not understood as a specific form of therapy and is not defined ideologically.

Client-centeredness rather means that a therapist adjusts his offers, goals, strategies, and interventions to a client in such a way that they can benefit optimally from the therapy.

"Client-centeredness" in this sense thus appears to be a necessary condition for psychotherapy.

References

Heckhausen, H. (1969). Förderung der Lernmotivierung und der intellektuellen Tüchtigkeit. In Roth, H. (Eds.), *Begabung und Lernen. Ergebnisse und Folgerungen neuer Forschungen, 193–228*. Klett.

20

Edge of the Possible

A therapist should promote the client's process and must therefore also challenge the client, but should not overwhelm them. Therefore, it is necessary for therapists to work as often as possible "at the edge of the possible". In doing so, they must assess where this edge is at any given time. Strategies are discussed with which a therapist can determine this.

From the principle of fit, it also results that *the level of difficulty of therapeutic interventions should absolutely be adapted to the client:* An intervention must be implemented by the client, and for this, a client must be capable.

Interventions should not overwhelm the client, because otherwise the therapy process stagnates, and probably the therapist-client relationship also deteriorates.

Interventions should also not *underchallenge* the client, because otherwise the therapy does not fully exploit the therapeutic potential: It thus becomes significantly less effective than it could be (cf. Sachse, 1992, 2003).

From these considerations, the therapeutic principle arises to work with a client as often as possible *"at the edge of the possible"*. That is, a therapist should *promote* the client through interventions, i.e., initiate new processes, manage difficult processes, etc., so that a client works as well as possible in the process. But a therapist should also not *overwhelm* a client, i.e., he should not implement interventions that a client cannot carry out.

R. Sachse, *Basic Psychological Insights for Psychotherapy*,
https://doi.org/10.1007/978-3-662-69780-1_20

A therapist should therefore always ask himself:

- What is the current "state of knowledge" of the client and which interventions lead the client further?
- Which current process goals (see below) can the therapist currently target with this client?
- How strongly is a client currently avoiding and which interventions reduce the avoidance?
- How strongly self-esteem burdening are the currently discussed contents and through which interventions can the client face them?

And the therapist should adapt flexibly to this.

The therapist should of course also always think about what assistance he can give a client so that he can carry out a difficult intervention: e.g., in the form of explanations, exercises, detailed instructions, motivations, instilling confidence, etc.

> A therapeutic *working at the edge of the possible* always requires that a therapist (based on his client model and his process model, see below) forms a hypothesis about what a client should implement and what he can implement.

A therapist should make it clear, however, *that the question of where the edge of the possible is, is always an empirical question:* The therapist only knows it when he has tried it out and analyzed what happens.

He should therefore bring the client to the edge of the possible and perceive what the client is currently doing.

As long as the edge of the possible is not reached, the client behaves cooperatively.

However, once the edge of the possible is reached, *avoidances set in:* A therapist recognizes these by *avoidance indicators,* such as "I don't know", answering questions that the therapist did not ask, changing topics, etc. (cf. Sachse, 1992, 2003).

If the therapist recognizes this, it makes sense to

- keep the client *there,* i.e., deal constructively with the avoidance, allow the client to leave the area again, but always bring him back;
- not to allow the client to completely avoid the area or to evade into "harmless" areas, because this can prevent the actually relevant, "hot" area from being clarified or worked on;

- but also not to *force* the client to continue into the aversive area, because this can make the therapy aversive for the client, strongly reinforce the avoidance behavior, lead to reactance and/or worsen the therapist-client relationship.

Doing this, however, requires a high level of expertise from the therapist.

References

Sachse, R. (1992). *Zielorientierte Gesprächspsychotherapie—Eine grundlegende Neukonzeption*. Hogrefe.
Sachse, R. (2003). *Klärungsorientierte Psychotherapie*. Hogrefe.

21

Motivation

It can be assumed that the most relevant client variable for predicting therapy success is the client's motivation for change. It is explained what is psychologically understood by "motivation for change" and how a therapist can promote this motivation.

In order to engage in change processes at all, to confront unpleasant content, implement therapeutic interventions, carry out strenuous processes, etc., a client must be *motivated.* Motivation processes on the client's side and motivation-promoting interventions on the therapist's side are of great importance in the psychotherapy process (cf. Sachse & Langens, 2015; Sachse et al. 2012, 2018).

And this is something a therapist should always keep in mind: A client can be very motivated, he can have decided to tackle problems, face difficulties and make an effort. But a client can also have the attitude of not doing more than is comfortable, or letting the therapist do the work.

Overview

Therefore, motivation is essential for constructive therapy processes, and without motivation, there can be no therapy success.

Therefore, motivation processes play a crucial role in psychotherapy.

R. Sachse, *Basic Psychological Insights for Psychotherapy*,
https://doi.org/10.1007/978-3-662-69780-1_21

It must be assumed that the *extent of motivation for change*, that a client realizes in the therapy process, is a crucial predictor for therapy success.

It is of great importance to distinguish between therapy motivation and change motivation.

Therapy motivation arises when a client realizes that he has costs that he does not want: This creates "*suffering pressure*", *and that creates therapy motivation.*

Therapy motivation is, however, merely the motivation to "put one's butt in the therapy chair". But a client can also associate intentions with this that have nothing to do with change, e.g.

- he may want the therapist to solve the problem for him,
- he may seek therapy to have his views confirmed,
- or to have a pleasant relationship,
- or to "vent",
- or he may want the therapist to help him better manipulate his interaction partners, etc.

Change motivation, however, psychologically requires much more than that:

- The client must recognize that *he* is the one *creating* the problem (and not just "has" it),
- he must recognize that the causes lie with him or "in" him,
- he must take responsibility for it,
- from this he must draw the conclusion that *he* needs to change something if "something" is to change,
- he must take responsibility for this change,
- he must *decide* to actively do something about it.

One can naively assume that every client who comes to psychotherapy is also motivated to change. This may be the case with phobic clients, but it is by no means the case with clients with personality disorders (cf. Sachse, 2019).

So there are clients (typically those with personality disorders) who have little or no motivation for change at the beginning of therapy. *And if this is the case, then it is a task of the therapist in the process to develop a motivation for change.*

Change motivation is therefore not an "entry requirement" for psychotherapy, but a significant *process goal.*

There are very elaborate therapy techniques for promoting or building change motivation (see Sachse et al. 2012, 2018).

Change motivation is not an all-or-nothing phenomenon: It can vary in strength. On the other hand, therapeutic measures place *demands* on the client: The client is supposed to internalize the perspective, follow questions, dispute schemas, etc. These demands are *differently difficult* for clients, differently strenuous, differently aversive, etc.; i.e. to realize the respective tasks, *a client needs different extents of change motivation.*

At the beginning of therapy, the demands can be relatively low, the client is then cooperative and works well.

Then the therapist increases his demands, and suddenly the client no longer cooperates. In phase 1, the motivation for change is greater than the demands—there is no problem.

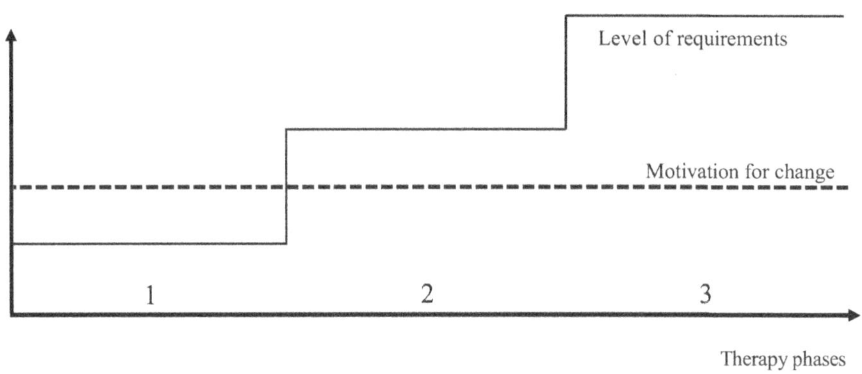

In Phase 2, however, the requirements are greater than the motivation to change: The client is no longer sufficiently motivated to carry out the processes.

If a client appears to have sufficient motivation to change in a phase, a therapist cannot assume that this will continue to be the case.

Therefore, a therapist should always keep an eye on the respective extent of a client's motivation to change, and he should (if necessary) take measures to increase the motivation to change.

References

Sachse, R. (2019). *Persönlichkeitsstörungen* (3rd ed.). Hogrefe.

Sachse, R., & Langens, T. A. (2015). Motivierung von Klienten im Therapieprozess: Herstellung und Steigerung von Änderungsmotivation. In R. Sachse, S. Schirm, & S. Kiszkenow-Bäker (Eds.), *Klärungsorientierte Psychotherapie in der Praxis*, 97–110. Pabst.

Sachse, R., Langens, T. A., & Sachse, M. (2012). *Klienten motivieren—Therapeutische Strategien zur Stärkung der Änderungsbereitschaft*. Psychiatrie-Verlag.

Sachse, R., Langens, T. A., & Sachse, M. (2018). *Klienten motivieren* (2nd. ed.). Psychiatrie-Verlag.

22

Planning and Flexibility

A therapist should develop a concept about which aspects on the client's side should be changed, i.e., he must realize a certain degree of planning. On the other hand, a therapist must still remain flexible in the face of more complex problems from clients. It is discussed how these aspects can be reconciled therapeutically.

Some of the considerations presented require a careful reconsideration of the topic of "therapy planning" and the flexibility of therapists.

These are primarily the following insights:

- A therapist does have a certain influence on the client's process, but he can never determine this process; everything that is possible can also happen in the therapy process and some of it is not only uncontrollable, but also unpredictable.
  The assumption that a therapist has the process under control, especially in the long term, is not tenable.
- Clients with high interactional mistrust will very likely not disclose the truly relevant problems to the therapist at the beginning of therapy.
  They will present less relevant problems or partial problems. And only when the therapist has succeeded in building trust will the clients address the *actual problems,* which should be the central focus.
  Therefore, topics can change in the process, but:

R. Sachse, *Basic Psychological Insights for Psychotherapy*,
https://doi.org/10.1007/978-3-662-69780-1_22

- sometimes this means that a client brings up less relevant topics; a therapist should not go along with this;
- sometimes a client also switches to (much) more important topics, and then the therapist should follow the client flexibly.

Since clients are highly likely not to disclose the relevant topics at the beginning of therapy, it is fundamentally impossible to derive reliable planning from the data that a therapist gains in the first five (to ten) hours.

With such clients, the "actual" problems emerge in the process as the client's trust in the therapist increases, often rather "incidentally".

When clients switch from less relevant to truly relevant problems, they also change the topic.

If a therapist has made a therapy plan based on initial information (which is nonsensical), *he should at least be able to adapt it to the new relevant topics.* Due to the described client situation, a therapist should definitely be *flexible*, especially since all client models are ultimately *hypotheses* and not immovable truths!

If the therapist then "carries out his planning anyway", he ignores highly relevant client information: The therapist is then in no way "client-appropriate", rather *he then treats past the client.*

- From the fact that many clients show a high degree of alienation at the beginning of therapy, i.e., they do not even know their central motives (see below), it follows that therapy goals can only be defined very provisionally at the beginning of therapy, if at all.
  If the alienation decreases during the course of therapy and a client can *then* define truly relevant therapy goals, a therapist should be able to be flexible again and adjust to the new, relevant therapy goals.

For these reasons, the following applies to therapy:

- At least with complex problems, a therapist cannot form fixed therapy plans at the beginning of therapy, as he will then "carry out the therapy".
- *Even if a therapist creates a therapy plan, it must always remain flexible and always be adapted to the client.* Therefore, a therapist should remain flexible, especially when working with clients who have more than one phobia, and that's why I (unlike Vogel and Schulte (1997)) would like to call

the opposite of planning "flexibility" and not "improvisation". Because a "flexible response" must always be thoughtful, it must be derived from the therapist's model and knowledge—and in my opinion, the term "improvisation" does not make this clear at all.

This, however, puts the therapist in a state of tension:

- On the one hand, he should derive strategies and interventions from his current model, because he should give the process *structure* (since the client cannot do this alone).
- He should also always define *process goals* that he is currently pursuing, because this also creates *structure.*
- But he should always view his model and its implications as hypotheses that need to be elaborated or revised by new client data.
- Flexibility then means,
  - to change the client model for a reason,
  - to derive new goals,
  - to develop new interventions and strategies.

Of course, a therapist should have a *plan*: This structures their actions and thus the process. *But the plan should function as a hypothesis, not as a law. The therapist must constantly rethink, modify, or possibly completely remake a plan!* And the plan should primarily include *process goals* (see below) and thus be more of a "medium-range" plan.

The assumption that a therapist should not be flexible can possibly be justified in the case of phobias, but certainly not for more complex disorders, which require more complex therapy processes to resolve.

Of course, a therapist should not arbitrarily change a plan: *It is necessary to consistently pursue relevant processes, topics, etc. for a considerable period of time, because processes always take time, and there is no alternative to this.*

If I, as a therapist, want to clarify or work on a schema with the client, this can only be achieved if it is worked on *consistently* for a period of time: Otherwise, the process deteriorates. *In doing so, a therapist is precisely pursuing process goals, and they know that they must continually "steer back" clients who often "go off track" into the process.*

The opposite of planning is not *chaos:* Of course, a therapist must repeatedly act according to a plan: However, they never know in advance *how long their plan is sensible* or when it needs to be modified or revised.

In any case, the assumption that one forms a plan at the beginning of therapy and can then follow it until the end of therapy is not sustainable from a psychological perspective, at least not if one wants to work in a client-centered manner.

References

Vogel, G., & Schulte, D. (1997). Methoden- und verlaufsorientierte Strategien von Psychotherapeuten. *Zeitschrift für Klinische Psychologie, 26*(1), 38–49.

23

Process Goals

A therapist should define so-called "process goals", i.e., goals that are now possible in the process and should be achieved as prerequisites for further client processes.

The therapist is here, as often, in a *dilemma:* On the one hand, he needs *goals,* to which he can align the therapy, on the other hand, the process cannot really be planned.

A possible solution to this dilemma is to *define process goals.*

A *process goal* is a goal that refers to a *specific process state* that a therapist wants to achieve next.

If a client shows high interactional mistrust, then the process goal is to build sufficient trust.

If the client's motivation to change is not sufficient, the process goal is to build sufficient motivation to change.

If a client has problems with an internal perspective, the process goal is to convey this strategy to the client.

As can be seen, process goals are not defined in terms of content, but by "psychological states or skills of a client".

R. Sachse, *Basic Psychological Insights for Psychotherapy*,
https://doi.org/10.1007/978-3-662-69780-1_23

Such process goals structure the therapist's actions to a great extent: The therapist is clear that he can only achieve the goal if he works consistently with the client for a while. However, the therapist is also clear that the path to it is *not linear:* He knows that the client repeatedly "gets off track", that he as a therapist must repeatedly recognize this and must repeatedly restart his strategy.

Thus, process goals define different therapy phases, and they structure a therapist's processing and action processes to a great extent—they are thus an *"inner GPS".*

Defining goals not in terms of content, but according to process states, has advantages: Clients must go through certain processes in a certain order so that each phase creates the prerequisite for the next phase. Therefore, one can generally define the phases, but one must assume that,

- not all clients have to go through all phases (as stated, phobics usually do not need a relationship design phase),
- not all clients go through the phases at the same speed
- or in the same way
- and require different sub-processes and different interventions from therapists,
- that the process flow is not linear, but some clients go through the phase several times (the process is thus *recursive*).

24

Responsibility

Both therapists and clients bear responsibility for the therapy process. The therapist's responsibility lies primarily in constructive process control, while the client's responsibility lies in engaging in processes, carrying them out, and implementing therapeutic insights.

This brings us to the topic of *responsibility:* Apparently, a therapist has a very high degree of *responsibility for constructively guiding the client process.* He should have as high an *expertise* as possible to be able to adapt well to all aspects of the process.

Overview

Ultimately, however, it is always the client who carries out the process: *A therapist can guide the client process, but cannot do it!*

It is always the client who carries out and must carry out the process: He must clarify his content, engage in disputations, test and modify new actions in reality, etc., if and when he wants to solve his problems!

The clarification and change processes take place "in" the client: In his psychological system, the client must carry them out. The therapist cannot perform these processes for the client. The client must *actively work: Therapeutic change is always hard work for a client!*

Psychotherapy means confronting unpleasant aspects of the self, actively carrying out processes, implementing the therapist's interventions, etc.

R. Sachse, *Basic Psychological Insights for Psychotherapy*,
https://doi.org/10.1007/978-3-662-69780-1_24

Psychotherapy is therefore always hard work, often unpleasant, aversive, conflict-ridden. It is never a "wellness event".

From what has been said, it is clear that both participants in the process, therapist and client, *each bear a part of the responsibility:*

- The therapist is responsible for good process control.
- The client is responsible for the content, i.e., for implementing therapeutic interventions, clarifying, etc.

Thus, it is quite obvious that the success of therapy is never dependent only on the therapist: It depends on both the therapist and the client.

A client can very well decide *not* to change and *not* to implement therapeutic interventions.

For clients, it is extremely easy to *"trip up a therapist"!*

If a client does not cooperate in the process, the therapist has means to motivate the client. If these do not work, a therapist may have to accept that a client does not want to change: This is ultimately the client's decision!

If a therapy does not "work", a therapist must always ask himself: "Have I worked lege artis?" or "Have I done my very best?" If he can answer these questions with "yes", he does not have to take responsibility for the failure of the therapy.

Overview

Thus, both the therapist and the client bear responsibility for the success of psychotherapy!

The therapist, as a *process expert,* has responsibility for constructive control, while the client, as a *content expert,* has the responsibility to actually carry out the processes.

25

Expertise, Expertise, Again and Again Expertise

> If a therapist wants to manage the complex tasks of psychotherapy, they require a high degree of *expertise.* Here, we will discuss what can be understood as expertise, how expertise is developed, and why it is so extremely relevant.

At many points in the book, we have come to the conclusion that therapists, if they want to practice a complex form of therapy with complex problems and complex clients, need a very high level of *expertise* (see Gäßler & Sachse, 1992a, b; Sachse, 1992a, b, 1994, 1996, 2006, 2009, 2022; Sachse et al., 2012).

Therefore, at this point, we will elaborate on what is meant by expertise, how expertise works, and why exactly a therapist needs expertise.

25.1 What is Expertise?

Expertise is a specific mental state of a person, characterized by special knowledge, special skills and abilities, special competencies, and which enables a person to handle tasks and problems in a specific performance area (a "performance domain") particularly quickly, particularly safely, and particularly effectively (cf. Ericsson, 1996, 2002, 2006a, b; Ericsson et al., 1993, 2006; Ericsson & Lehmann, 1996; Ericsson & Smith, 1991; Zimmerman, 2006).

R. Sachse, *Basic Psychological Insights for Psychotherapy*,
https://doi.org/10.1007/978-3-662-69780-1_25

What distinguishes experts can be compared primarily with so-called "novices", i.e., people who work in the same domain (e.g., psychotherapy) but who do not yet have a high level of competence.

Experts are characterized by the following:

- Experts have a significantly higher level of knowledge than novices.
- This primarily refers to *action-relevant knowledge.*
- The knowledge of experts is significantly better structured, more accessible, and available than that of novices.
- The knowledge of experts is organized more prototypically, it is organized as it is actually needed for problem-solving and decision-making.
- Experts not only have knowledge about phenomena (e.g., diagnoses) but especially knowledge about how these actually manifest in reality (knowing a diagnosis does not mean that one can draw correct conclusions from data!).
- Experts are able to quickly *establish patterns and relationships,* they quickly develop good hypotheses and can test, validate, etc. them well.
- *And above all: Experts can distinguish much faster, more securely, and more validly between relevant and irrelevant information.*As a result, they store relevant information and do not "clog" their processing and storage with irrelevant information!
- Experts can simplify complex problems by quickly recognizing the really important aspects and being able to focus on them.
- Experts can process a lot of information "automatically", which allows them to process much more information "in parallel" than novices.
- Experts can flexibly switch between different information areas, so that they can, for example, "monitor" different process aspects in the therapy process.
- Experts can draw much faster and much more valid conclusions from data than novices.
- Experts can work specifically in an "intuitive-holistic processing mode": As a result, they perceive implicit information such as facial expressions, etc. much better than novices.
- Experts store information differently than novices: They form structures, meta-propositions, establish connections, focus on relevant aspects, etc. They thus form far better and more effective client models than novices in a much shorter time.
- Because of these facts, experts can make much faster and much more valid decisions than novices.
- Experts have sophisticated processing and action strategies.

- Experts can think far ahead and anticipate possibilities and problems much better than novices.
- Experts can monitor their actions better and react more flexibly than novices.

However, all these considerations lead to another essential consequence: The information base underlying a therapist's expertise should be as well structured and thus as consistent, networked, etc. as possible. This has the consequence for therapy training that beginners should not simply be taught many therapy methods "side by side" or concepts that do not correspond at all, but that it is important to *connect*and integrate the information. Twenty seminars on very different concepts do not create high expertise! Even if all seminars are held by highly competent lecturers: This rather creates a pile of unstructured knowledge.

25.2 Why is expertise important?

It is completely evident in expertise research, *that a person requires a higher level of expertise, the more complex the requirements are.*

If a person needs to process information quickly, make decisions quickly, act effectively quickly, etc., then they can only do this with a high level of expertise.

As we have clearly seen in the previous chapters, complex psychotherapy with complex problems and complex clients places exactly such high demands on the therapist.

A therapist must, for example,

- process the information "incoming" from the client "in real time",
- even when this information is "encoded", poorly structured, idiosyncratic, etc.,
- quickly draw conclusions from the data, form hypotheses,
- "hold these hypotheses in suspense", test, validate, elaborate, etc.,
- he must form a client and process model based on this and constantly update these models,
- he must make therapeutic decisions quickly and confidently,
- he must have elaborate and flexible action strategies,
- which he can convert into good, effective interventions,
- he must always monitor, evaluate and respond to the effects of his interventions, etc. etc.

25.3 How is expertise developed?

To develop expertise, one must first build a comprehensive and well-structured *knowledge base*. This is done through literature, seminars, etc.

However, this alone is by no means sufficient for the development of high expertise.

To develop expertise, one needs so-called *"reflective practice":* One must

- implement processing and actions in *practice*,
- repeatedly look at and reflect on an action,
- discover mistakes, confront mistakes and learn from mistakes,
- continually improve one's actions, processing, etc., and
- test again in practice.
- And: The whole thing again, again and again.

Expertise research assumes that to become an expert, *10,000 h (!)* of training and another 1000 h of reflection are needed: with a supervisor, a guide, etc.

Walter Kintsch puts it this way: "An expert is a person, who does the right things at the right time. But: It takes 10 years of hard training to become an expert."

"Ten years of hard training" means, for example,

- that one is by no means an expert based on a predominantly theoretical education,
- that one is not an expert even after 2–3 years of practice,
- that one is not an expert if one predominantly has theoretical knowledge,
- that one must continually train and reflect and train, etc.,
- that the fact that one has been working in a domain for 10 years *does not* guarantee that one is an expert (!!!),
- that one exhibits a higher level of expertise, the more demanding and complex the domain in which one has trained.

Less demanding domains therefore only lead to limited expertise! In the domain areas in which one is not trained, one logically does not have any expertise.

And therefore it is not surprising that therapists cannot do certain things if they have not been trained in them: If you do not learn to analyze client processes, you cannot assess processes. If you do not learn to recognize relationship messages, manipulations, etc., you cannot do that either!

And this also means: If a sample of therapists cannot do something specific, one cannot *conclude from this that therapists generally cannot do this, but only that therapists with this specific expertise cannot do it!*

References

Ericsson, K. A. (1996). The acquisition of expert performance: An introduction to some of the issues. In K. A. Ericsson (Eds.), *The road to excellence: The acquisition of expert performance in the arts and sciences, sports, and games* (pp. 1–50). Erlbaum.

Ericsson, K. A. (2002). Attaining excellence through deliberate practice: Insights from the study of expert performance. In M. Ferrari (Eds.), *The pursuit of excellence in education* (pp. 21–55). Erlbaum.

Ericsson, K. A. (2006a). An introduction to the Cambridge handbook of expertise and expert performance: Its development, organization, and content. In K. A. Ericsson, N. Charness, P. J. Feltovich, & R. R. Hoffmann (Eds.), *The Cambridge handbook of expertise and expert performance* (pp. 3–20). University Press.

Ericsson, K. A. (2006b). The influence of expertice and deliberate practice on the development of superior expert performance. In K. A. Ericsson, N. Charness, P. J. Feltovich, & R. R. Hoffman (Eds.), *The Cambridge handbook of expertise and expert performance* (pp. 653–682). University Press.

Ericsson, K. A., & Smith, J. (1991). *Toward a general theory of expertise. Prospects and limits.* Cambridge University Press.

Ericsson, K. A., & Lehmann, A. C. (1996). Expert and exceptional performance: Evidence on maximal adaptations on task constraints. *Annual Review of Psychology, 47,* 273–305.

Ericsson, K. A., Krampe, R. T., & Tesch-Römer, C. (1993). The role of deliberate practice in the acquisition of expert performance. *Psychological Review, 100,* 363–406.

Ericsson, K. A., Charness, N., Feltovich, P. J., & Hoffman, R. R. (2006). *The Cambridge Hanndbook of Expertise and Expert Performance.* University Press.

Gäßler, B., & Sachse, R. (1992a). Psychotherapeuten als Experten: Unter welchen Voraussetzungen können Psychotherapeuten die komplexe sprachliche Information ihrer Klienten verarbeiten? In R. Sachse, G. Lietaer, & W. B. Stiles (Eds.), *Neue Handlungskonzepte der Klientenzentrierten Psychotherapie* (S. 133–142). Asanger.

Gäßler, B. & Sachse, R. (1992b). Psychotherapeuten als Experten. In L. Montada (Eds.), *Bericht über den 38. Kongress der Deutschen Gesellschaft für Psychologie in Trier, 1,* 663–664. Hogrefe.

Sachse, R. (1992a). *Zielorientierte Gesprächspsychotherapie—Eine grundlegende Neukonzeption.* Hogrefe.

Sachse, R. (1992b). Psychotherapie als komplexe Aufgabe: Verarbeitungs-, Intentionsbildungs- und Handlungsplanungsprozesse bei Psychotherapeuten. In R. Sachse, G. Lietaer, & W. B. Stiles (Eds.), *Neue Handlungskonzepte der Klientenzentrierten Psychotherapie* (pp. 109–112). Asanger.

Sachse, R. (1994). Der Einfluß von Expertise und Lageorientierung auf den Informationsverarbeitungsprozeß von Therapeuten. In K. Pawlik (Eds.), *39. Kongress der Deutschen Gesellschaft für Psychologie, 601*. Psychologisches Institut I der Universität Hamburg.

Sachse, R. (1996). *Auswirkungen von Expertise und Handlungsorientierung von Therapeuten auf die Elaboration von Klientenmodellen.* Berichte aus der Arbeitseinheit Klinische Psychologie: Ruhr-Universität Bochum.

Sachse, R. (2006). Psychotherapie-Ausbildung aus der Sicht der Expertise-Forschung. In R. Sachse & P. Schlebusch (Eds.), *Perspektiven Klärungsorientierter Psychotherapie* (pp. 306–324). Pabst.

Sachse, R. (2009). Psychotherapeuten als Experten. In R. Sachse, J. Fasbender, J. Breil, & O. Püschel (Eds.), *Grundlagen und Konzepte Klärungsorientierter Psychotherapie* (pp. 269–291). Hogrefe.

Sachse, R. (2022). *Komplexität in der Psychotherapie.* Hogrefe.

Sachse, R., Fasbender, J., & Hammelstein, P. (2012). Wie sollte eine Ausbildung in Psychotherapie beschaffen sein? *Report Psychologie, 2,* 50–53.

Zimmerman, B. J. (2006). Development and adaptation of expertise: The role of self-regulatory processes and beliefs. In K. A. Ericsson, N. Charness, P. J. Feltovich, & R. R. Hoffman (Eds.), *The Cambridge handbook of expertise and expert performance* (pp. 705–722). University Press.

26

Didacticization

Sometimes it is necessary for a therapist to explain the therapeutic approach to a client: This is referred to as "didacticization". Here, principles are outlined that a therapist should follow.

In some cases, it is useful for a therapist to provide information to the client, explain aspects, clarify procedures, etc.

Such an approach can be referred to as *didacticization.*

According to Fiedler's considerations, didacticizations should only be implemented under two conditions:

1. The client *wants* certain information, expects explanations, etc.
2. The therapist concludes that the client needs information, explanations, etc. *needs.*

If a client wants information, it is their right to receive it: Therefore, it should definitely be conveyed to the client.

However, the therapist can also didacticize because he comes to the conclusion,

- that a client lacks essential information, which he needs to understand interventions, develop motivation, etc.,
- that a client needs specific instructions for a method, such as when introducing a "one-person role play",

R. Sachse, *Basic Psychological Insights for Psychotherapy*,
https://doi.org/10.1007/978-3-662-69780-1_26

- that the client needs to understand how his disorder works and how he can better adjust to it, e.g. in the case of borderline clients,
- that the client has *misconceptions* that hinder therapy and should therefore be addressed by the therapist.

Thus, a therapist must convey to the client, for example,

- that psychotherapy requires active participation from the client, that the success of therapy also depends on this,
- that a therapist cannot solve the client's problems for the client,
- but that he can only actively help with the solution,
- that the therapist cannot perform magic or that he is not a "savior",
- that the therapist's task cannot be to stabilize the client's problem, etc. etc.

If a therapist implements a didacticization, he should adhere to certain psychological principles:

- The therapist should give explanations *as briefly as possible*—if he does not, he overloads the client's processing capacity and the client "switches off". Therapists should therefore not give lectures, but only convey to the client exactly what he should know, and no more.
- The therapist should give his explanations as clearly, precisely and concisely as possible: He should *explicitly* say what he means or what he wants. He should not communicate indirectly, "through the flower".
- The therapist's explanations should be as easy to understand as possible, so:
  - short sentences,
  - simple grammar,
  - slow speaking,
  - take breaks, give the client time to process, etc.
- The therapist should adapt his explanations to the intellectual and educational level of the client.
- The therapist should, if possible, *anchor what he wants to convey in the client's concrete experiential background*: He should, for example, use metaphors from the client's areas of life, establish connections to the client's concrete experiences, etc.

This makes it easier for the client to understand the intended meaning and apply it to themselves.

Part III

Basic Psychological Insights on the Client's Sid

Of course, it is of central importance that clients in psychotherapy clarify, work on, and solve their individual problems.

In the therapeutic analysis of these problems, however, it is repeatedly noticed that these, at least in part, are due to unfavorable and sometimes incorrect basic assumptions of the individuals.

If that is the case, then it seems sensible to impart specific psychological knowledge to a client so that they can solve their problems sustainably and, above all, prevent the development of new problems. Or it may be useful to convey these insights to clients in the process, for example, through a "Socratic dialogue".

27

Avoidance Preserves the Problem

> Clients must recognize that avoiding problems actually stabilizes them and makes them unsolvable. If you want to solve a problem, you have to face it, and that requires making a decision.

Clients often believe they can solve a problem by not confronting it.

Of course, avoidance has immediate positive consequences (in the sense of a C-): If I avoid problems, I avoid aversive states, I avoid the perception that I apparently cannot solve something, I avoid negative emotions when I do not confront self-esteem burdening schemas, etc.

A therapist must make it clear to the client, both through interventions and brief didactic explanations, that while avoidance leads to C- in the short term, it generates high costs in the long term.

No matter whether a phobic person avoids heights or a personality-disordered client avoids certain schemas—the rule always applies: *Avoidance preserves the problem!*

In principle, you can only solve a problem if you "face it", perceive it as a problem, consider it, analyze it, etc.

The client should therefore recognize that he can only solve a problem if he

- recognizes and acknowledges that he has a problem,
- confronts the problem,
- is willing to *face all aspects of the problem,* no matter how unpleasant and burdensome they may be.

R. Sachse, *Basic Psychological Insights for Psychotherapy*,
https://doi.org/10.1007/978-3-662-69780-1_27

Many clients only slowly recognize this in the course of the therapy process, and they only stop avoiding when they

- have trust in the therapist,
- have trust in themselves, e.g. that they can endure certain states or cope with problems,
- when the therapist has made it clear *that* they avoid and *how* they avoid,
- when they recognize that this effectively hinders problem solving.

The therapeutic consequences are:

- Therapists may need to provide didactic explanations to convey relevant psychological aspects to clients.
- Therapists should confront clients with avoidance.
- Therapists should systematically work on the client's avoidances: There are elaborate procedures for this (see Sachse et al., 2011).

References

Sachse, R., Fasbender, J., & Sachse, M. (2011). Die Bearbeitung von Vermeidung in der Klärungsorientierten Psychotherapie. In R. Sachse, J. Fasbender, J. Breil, & M. Sachse (Eds.), *Perspektiven Klärungsorientierter Psychotherapie II* (pp. 156–183). Pabst.

28

Dealing with Risks

Sometimes clients are afraid to take risks. However, every change implies risks, and such fears should be therapeutically addressed.

It is a fundamental realization that no person can eliminate or control all risks in their life.

Every person has only a relatively small degree of control over their life.

For example, they cannot control

- what interaction partners will do next,
- which conflicts, problems, etc. will arise or when,
- whether they will be hit by a car, robbed, frustrated, etc.,
- whether a meteorite will strike them, etc.

Often, one can make *rough risk assessments based on one's own knowledge and experiences, but this is only successful in terms of rough probability estimates: Conflicts with partners are much more likely than meteorite strikes.*

R. Sachse, *Basic Psychological Insights for Psychotherapy*,
https://doi.org/10.1007/978-3-662-69780-1_28

Overview

Based on such rough probability estimates, *one can roughly calculate risks and thus avoid decisions with high risk.*

But as a human being, one can never reduce a risk to zero! Something like absolute safety or complete control is fundamentally unachievable.

One must live with this realization as a human being, unless one compensates for it through self-deception (cf. Sachse, 2020).

However, there are clients who find this difficult and who want to avoid risks at all costs. These are, for example, clients with a high need for control, obsessive-compulsive personality disorder, generalized anxiety disorder, or people who are afraid of making wrong decisions because they could trigger "disasters".

Such an intention to "achieve safety" usually leads to

- great concern,
- massive control actions,
- restriction of the range of behavior,
- difficult decisions leading to decision paralysis.

And thus, the attempt to avoid risks usually exacerbates the problem or at least stabilizes it!

Based on these considerations, a client in therapy should recognize

- that one can *never* reduce risks to zero,
- but one can learn to estimate risks,
- that such estimates can always only be made with a certain probability, never with certainty,
- *that every decision carries risks,*
- that one can only estimate risks up to a certain point,
- that beyond this, further analyses are not useful and only hinder the decision.

As a human being, if one wants to live meaningfully in the real world, one must accept that there are always risks and one can never completely avoid risks.

An attitude that can be useful here has been formulated by Lee Child in his "Reacher" novels: "Hope for the best and be prepared for the worst."

The therapeutic consequences are:

- Often didacticization: The therapist explains the psychological backgrounds to the client.
- The therapist makes the search for security transparent and confronts the client with it and with the resulting costs.
- A therapist addresses the psychological reasons for such a high need for security.

References

Sachse, R. (2020). *Die Psychologie der Selbsttäuschung*. Springer.

29

Decisions

Clients may have trouble making decisions for various reasons, which can significantly affect their quality of life. Therefore, therapists should pay special attention to this aspect.

We all constantly make decisions: In the restaurant, we decide what we want to eat, we decide where to go on vacation, which car to buy, which apartment to move into, which profession to choose, and with which partner to spend our lives.

Many of the decisions we make are of little relevance: Choosing schnitzel over goulash in a restaurant can be annoying if the schnitzel is bad, but it has no lasting consequences.

However, some decisions are of existential importance: The partner I choose (and against whom I decide) can determine my future life to an extremely high degree. The profession I choose has a decisive influence on my entire life design. Therefore, decisions play a crucial role in people's lives.

29.1 What is a Decision?

Making a decision means *that you now want something specific:* You now want to pursue a goal, do something specific, achieve, avoid, etc..

R. Sachse, *Basic Psychological Insights for Psychotherapy*,
https://doi.org/10.1007/978-3-662-69780-1_29

You *decide* to invest some time and effort, to strive, to "stick with it", to make an effort, to solve problems that stand in your way, etc. (see the so-called "Rubicon model by Heckhausen et al., 1987; see also: Sachse, 2020a).

"Decision" means to move from the state of "I want" to the state of "I will": This gives the person "power", they are determined to do something specific, to achieve goals, they are determined to do something for it, to face problems, to be disciplined, to forego alternatives, etc. (see Kuhl, 1983, 1994, 2001).

In the case of relevant decisions, a person wants to make such a decision *that they can stick with for a long time, "that they can stand behind", "that is okay for them".*

And therefore, the person needs a decision that (over time) *brings more gains than costs:* It can be exhausting and sometimes frustrating to stick with a decision (costs), but in the long run, it has to be worth it (gains) or one must be able to expect gains.

To Make a Sustainable Decision, it Must Meet *Two*Criteria

- It should be *rationally thought out,*so that it is highly likely to work "in reality".
- It must be compatible with one's own central ("implicit") motives, so that it leads to actions that can create a state of satisfaction.

This means: A rational "thinking through" of decisions is undoubtedly important: But it is not sufficient.

A central prerequisite for the "sustainability" of a decision is that the decision is compatible with central motives (see Gigerenzer, 2007a, b; Sachse et al., 2012, 2018).

You need to know what you want to achieve with the decision, and you need to know that it will personally do you good and make you satisfied. And, if possible, you should strive for exactly that.

This means that you can never make a decision *solely*based on rational criteria, but always also on affective criteria: The decision must feel "good and consistent".

To be able to make a decision, I therefore first need to find out for myself:

- What do I actually want?
- What is good for me?
- What makes me satisfied?

And also:

- What do I not want?
- What is not good for me?
- What makes me dissatisfied?

These are all questions about "motive compatibility": Does what I strive for, what I want, really correspond to important motives, and can the resulting action really create *satisfaction?*

If I can assess this, then there is a high probability that the effects I achieve will be positive for me in the short and especially in the long term: Then I have the impression again and again that the decision is okay. And that makes a decision *sustainable.*

> *To be able to make such a decision, I should therefore know my motives, desires, longings, goals, etc., and assess whether the decision can lead to the satisfaction of these aspects.* I should therefore have "access to my own motivation system" and thus not show any alienation.

This leads to the important realization that I can never make a (relevant!) decision based solely on rational criteria: *Of course, I must think through a decision rationally, asking myself questions like:*

- Can I achieve the goal?
- Do I have the competencies?
- Is the goal achievable in principle?
- Can it be achieved in the (social) context in which I live?
- What costs, problems, obstacles can occur?
- Can I overcome these? Etc.

Considering such aspects is important, as the decision should lead to actions and effects that work in my reality: that bring more gains than costs ("on the long run").

However, this is by no means sufficient for a sustainable decision: I must not only analyze whether the decision is "realistic", I must (above all) still decide whether it corresponds to my motives!

And that means: A decision must also be made according to emotional or (more precisely) affective aspects: It must not only be well thought out, it *must above all feel right* (cf. Sachse & Langens, 2014)!

Therapeutically, this means that a therapist should not only stimulate a client to a rational analysis and "think through" the decision. It means that the therapist should also guide the client to "let possible consequences affect him" in order to feel whether they "feel good".

29.2 Conflict and Decision

Many decisions are preceded by a *conflict.*

A *conflict* means that as a person you have more than one course of action, e.g. you have to decide between A and B. Both A and B now have certain advantages (gains), but also certain disadvantages (costs). With *every* decision, there is thus a 4-field matrix:

Alternative	Gains	Costs
A		
B		

With every decision, the person hopes to achieve certain gains that they believe are relevant to them.

Overview

But: It is also an important realization that *every decision involves costs.*

There are always *two* sources of costs:

- When a person decides for A, they often forego the gains that alternative B would offer them.
- When a person decides for A, it always has "side effects" that are less pleasant, sometimes it even implies high costs.

Every decision is, whether you want it or not, *always associated with risks and side effects!*

A decision is pending when the person

- cannot have both alternatives,
- so either only A or only B.

And then the person has the problem:

- A has certain advantages, and B has other advantages,
- if they decide for A, then they get the advantages of A,
- but at the same time they have to forego the advantages of B,
- both A and B are associated with certain disadvantages,
- if they decide for A, then they must also accept the disadvantages of A.

So the person must weigh up

- which advantages are more important to them personally: those of A or those of B,
- *with which costs they can live best:*with the disadvantages of A or those of B.

These considerations have some important psychological implications:

- The decision-making task is *highly complex:*Because the person must evaluate many positive aspects simultaneously and then come to an overall result of the type A > B.
- The same applies to negative aspects.
- The person must then weigh positive and negative aspects against each other.

> One implication is particularly important: *There is no decision without cost!*

If I have a choice between two possible partners and I choose partner A, then

- partner A will certainly have aspects that are personally important to me and more important than those of partner B, but partner A will always also have aspects that I like less or not at all, which I necessarily have to deal with by making the decision,
- I have to give up many positive aspects of partner B because A simply does not have them (that's exactly what makes B so attractive!).

These costs of a decision are fundamentally unavoidable!

And one must be clear that the person should have considered all these aspects in a decision in order for a decision to be sustainable! For this, a person should adopt an "intuitive-holistic mode" when making a decision in order to be able to weigh many aspects at the same time (cf. Sachse et al. 2018).

Many people make the mistake of wanting to believe that decisions only bring gains or should do so: They thus completely exclude the costs from their perception!

But they do not take into account the costs in their decision: The costs exist in reality, and when the person then lives with A, the disadvantages of A will become unmistakable after some time. This can become so serious that the person begins to question the decision and *falls into a conflict again:* But this proves that the original decision was not sustainable!

However, one must see that something like this can *always* happen in principle, as one can never fully estimate consequences, especially long-term ones (see the aspect "risks"). But in the therapy process, it is about taking into account everything that can be estimated at the moment, *in order to make the decision as sustainable as possible.*

Unfortunately, there is *not* only the decision between two predominantly positive alternatives: Sometimes one also has to decide between alternatives that both generate costs, and of different kinds. In this case, the decisive question is not:

- Which decision brings me the greatest benefit? Instead, the question is:
- With which costs can I live better?

29.3 You Cannot Not Decide

Many clients believe that they cannot make a decision, and that this solves their problem.

Psychologically, however, one must see that one cannot not decide.

As a person, in relation to a problem, one always has at least *two* alternatives:

- One can decide to tackle the problem and solve it.
- Or one can decide not to tackle it.

Clients then believe (or *want* to believe) that it will get better if they do not make a decision, *as if there were a third alternative* (which solves everything and costs nothing), but unfortunately there is not: The idea of such an alternative is based on self-deception (it is a kind of "magical thinking").

One must recognize: If a client does not decide, then he implicitly decides, whether he wants to or not, not to tackle the problem. Although he *seemingly* does not make a decision, he still makes a decision. *You cannot not decide!*

If the client seemingly does not make a decision, he also decides that everything remains as it is. Since many psychological problems tend to worsen, the client also decides to accept a worsening.

Since the client does not explicitly decide, *he also does not decide to accept the costs of the decision:* Instead, he "complains" about his costs and hopes that a *"savior"* will make them disappear (with the therapist often supposed to act as such a "savior").

A therapist should at some point *confront*the client with such ideas and their consequences: Because if the client *actively changes nothing,* then also *"itself"* changes nothing! We call such a confrontation the "*Alternatives-Confrontation*" (cf. Sachse, 2003).

Of course, a client can also decide to do nothing: But then he should be aware of the resulting consequences!

29.4 Decisions and Pseudo-Decisions

A person can make a decision and then "stand behind this decision": She no longer doubts it, implements it, etc.

If a person has a conflict of the kind where they must choose between Partner A and Partner B, they can make a viable and sustainable decision.

The dissonance theory has shown that a decision leads to systematically reducing dissonances (see Festinger, 1957; Frey & Gaska, 2001; Harmon-Jones & Harmon-Jones, 2002; Harmon-Jones & Mills, 1999; Peus et al., 2006): If one decides for A, then A now appears significantly more attractive than B and than before the decision, and B appears significantly worse than A and before the decision.

We refer to this as the "contrast effect": The system behaves as if the decision was evident and has always been evident.

Of course, this is a strategy of self-deception, but it is a so-called "positive illusion" (see Baumeister, 1989; Colvin & Block, 1994; Försterling & Morgenstern, 2006; Taylor & Brown, 1988): It clearly serves to stabilize a decision by defusing the conflict or believing that there is no conflict (and there never really was one).

This means: A real decision significantly reduces the conflict or often even makes it "conflict-free".

Thus, a central criterion for a client having made a "real" decision is the fact that they are conflict-free after a decision. If they are not conflict-free, they have not made a real decision!

Such conflict-freedom is essential, it is a so-called "positive self-deception" (Sachse, 2020b): *It is necessary to stabilize a decision.* A so-called "contrast effect" arises: After the decision, the aspects for the chosen alternative appear extremely positive and those for the non-chosen alternative extremely negative, and the person has the impression that this has "basically" always been evident (which is clearly not true).

However, there are also *"extrinsic" reasons*for making a decision: In the conflict between Partner A and Partner B, it is likely that this conflict will persist for a long time and create *a highly aversive state* for the person.

Then the person makes a decision for B, not because they really know and feel that this is the right decision, but only *because they want to escape the aversive state.*

However, this is not a "real decision" based on clear (rational and affective) criteria: It is an "extrinsic" decision, which merely serves to end a *aversive state* (thus achieving a C-).

*This does not make the person conflict-free in any way,*because the conflict is not resolved, but only avoided!

This type of decision can be called a *"pseudo-decision".*

Thus, a person who has to choose between Partner A and Partner B may "have had enough" and move to Partner B. This provides *short-term*relief, but soon the conflict resumes unabated.

So they move back to Partner A and so on and so forth.

And this action does not resolve the conflict, but exacerbates it on all levels.

A Therapist Recognizes a *Real Decision* by

- the client having intensively dealt with the pros and cons of each alternative,
- having conducted rational analyses,
- having especially "consulted" their affects,
- being *determined* after the decision to put it into action, to face problems,
- *and above all, being conflict-free after the decision.* This subjective conflict-freedom is essential; it is of course a self-deception, but a highly functional one!

A *pseudo-decision* can be recognized by the fact that it shows opposite effects:

- The client has not intensively dealt with the conflict aspects in the process. Above all, they have not taken note of their affects towards the decision.
- They are by no means determined to implement the decision (even against obstacles).
- And above all: They are not conflict-free after the decision: The conflict is still active and constantly questions the decision.
- The client is therefore unable to accept the costs incurred by the decision, but these constantly trigger new conflicts.

A therapist should recognize pseudo-decisions as such and confront the client with them.

The therapist should repeatedly "lead the client back into the conflict" and prompt them to confront it, to reflect on it again and again, until "the system tips": Then, after some time, the client can make a real decision.

Then they move out from A and into B, and this decision is no longer questioned.

Such a process can take some time and a therapist should repeatedly question pseudo-decisions, re-enter into a conflict resolution, until the system has come to a "real" decision.

It is very important to see here that a pseudo-decision ultimately does not benefit a client, indeed it often exacerbates the problem.

References

Baumeister, R. F. (1989). The optimal margin of illusion. *Journal of Social and Clinical Psychology, 8,* 176–189.

Colvin, C. R., & Block, J. (1994). Do positive illusions foster mental health? An examination of the Taylor and Brown formulation. *Psychological Bulletin, 116,* 3–20.

Festinger, L. (1957). *A theory of cognitive dissonance.* Stanford University Press.

Försterling, F., & Morgenstern, M. (2006). Positive Illusionen. In H.-W. Bierhoff & D. Frey (Eds.), *Handbuch der Sozialpsychologie und Kommunikationspsychologie* (pp. 363–372). Hogrefe.

Frey, D. & Gaska, A. (2001). Die Theorie der kognitiven Dissonanz. In: D. Frey & M. Irle (Eds.), *Theorien der Sozialpsychologie. Bd. 1: Kognitive Theorien,* (pp. 275–324). Huber.

Gigerenzer, G. (2007a). *Gut feelings: The Intelligence of the Unconscious.* Penguin.

Gigerenzer, G. (2007b). *Bauchentscheidungen: Die Intelligenz des Unbewussten und die Macht der Intuition.* C. Bertelsmann.

Harmon-Jones, E., & Harmon-Jones, C. (2002). Testing the action-based model of cognitive dissonance: The effect of action orientation on postdecisional attitudes. *Personality and Social Psychology Bulletin, 28,* 711–723.

Harmon-Jones, E., & Mills, J. (1999). *Cognitive dissonance: Progress on a pivotal theory in social psychology.* Science conference series.

Heckhausen, H., Gollwitzer, P. M., & Weinert, F. E. (1987). *Jenseits des Rubikon: Der Wille in den Humanwissenschaften.* Springer.

Kuhl, J. (1983). Emotion, Kognition und Motivation: I. Auf dem Wege zu einer systemtheoretischen Betrachtung der Emotionsgenese. *Sprache und Kognition, 2*(1), 1–27.

Kuhl, J. (1994). Handlungs- und Lageorientierung. In W. Sarges (Ed.), *Managementdiagnostik* (2. ed.). Hogrefe.

Kuhl, J. (2001). *Motivation und Persönlichkeit: Interaktionen psychischer Systeme.* Hogrefe.

Peus, C., Frey, D., & Stöger, H. (2006). Theorie der kognitiven Dissonanz. In H. W. Bierhoff & D. Frey (Eds.), *Handbuch der Sozialpsychologie und Kommunikationspsychologie* (pp. 373–379). Hogrefe.

Sachse, R. (2003). *Klärungsorientierte Psychotherapie.* Hogrefe.

Sachse, R. (2020a). *Selbstregulation und Selbstkontrolle.* Hogrefe.

Sachse, R. (2020b). *Die Psychologie der Selbsttäuschung.* Springer.

Sachse, R., Langens, T. A., & Sachse, M. (2012). *Klienten motivieren – Therapeutische Strategien zur Stärkung der Änderungsbereitschaft.* Psychiatrie-Verlag.

Sachse, R., Langens, T. A., & Sachse, M. (2018). *Klienten motivieren* (2. ed.). Psychiatrie-Verlag.

Taylor, S. E., & Brown, J. D. (1988). Illusion and well-being: A social psychological perspective on mental health. *Psychological Bulletin, 103,* 193–210.

30

Construction and Evaluation

People construct their reality based on "data" provided by their context. They then evaluate such constructions based on their motivation system. These are *two* different processes that clients often mix up. The difference should be made clear to clients.

30.1 Reality Models

People try to create a *"model of reality"*, that is, to understand "how reality works", and from this to create a *knowledge base* from which they can draw conclusions, which they can use to guide their decisions, etc.

It is important to understand how reality works, especially social reality: I need to have a model of what consequences I can expect with what probability from which behavior.

I need to develop a model about interaction partners, a knowledge about what they want, what they react positively to, where they are "allergic", etc.: Then and only then can I act purposefully, avoid actions with negative consequences and realize actions that are likely to have positive consequences (see the "Theory of mind" (Förstl, 2007)).

Such "reality models" are therefore of crucial importance if one wants to live successfully in reality and generate more gains than costs.

R. Sachse, *Basic Psychological Insights for Psychotherapy*,
https://doi.org/10.1007/978-3-662-69780-1_30

From an epistemological as well as psychological point of view, it is clear that people can never have a completely valid conception of reality (Baumann, 2015; Ernst, 2016; Gabriel, 2016; Grundmann, 2017).

Overview

There are no "self-explanatory facts" (this is a very common misconception). Strictly speaking, so-called "facts" are also already the result of interpretations. What appears to us as "facts" is always already the result of interpretation processes. Rather, there are "data" that are generated by certain observations and *that always have to be interpreted:* Such interpretations (and also observations) always depend on many factors, e.g. knowledge, preferences, schemas, self-deception, etc.

A person *"always constructs a reality"*, but: Some constructions work well in reality (= generate more gains than costs) and others do not work well, i.e. they generate more costs than gains.

Therefore, one can assume that there are interpretations that "validly" represent reality, that "work in reality", from which one can derive actions, for example, that bring gains. "Valid" in this context means "accurate"; however, there are very different criteria for validity. Here the criterion is that a construction allows conclusions and actions that "work", that is, produce more gains than costs overall.

Many interpretations, however, are invalid; the conclusions drawn from them lead to actions that create problems.

Accordingly, there are also valid, i.e. well-functioning reality models: The actions, decisions, etc. derived from them "work": They predominantly (never only!) produce positive effects. And of course, there are invalid models from which actions, etc. are derived that do not work.

From these considerations, one can draw a central conclusion: *Every assessment is a construction!* It is a construction that can be more or less valid, but it always remains a construction, a *hypothesis* about reality.

No person can know for sure how "reality" exactly works or what exactly is "real": Therefore, one can never say, "something *is* this or that way", that is the reality and it cannot be questioned.

But this means:

- *Every* assumption that the client makes, about themselves, about interaction partners, about social relationships, about partners, etc., is a *construction.*
- This can be more or less valid.
- Unfortunately, it can also be *very invalid*, i.e. it does not work well in reality and thus creates (massive) problems.
- *But this also means that every construction is fundamentally questionable.*
- It can be checked, tested, disputed, questioned.
- And it can and should be modifiable, so it should be elaborated, modified, specified or possibly completely discarded.

Psychologically, one can assume that people constantly test such hypotheses through their actions and that they learn from the effects: If they receive negative feedback, they can question their assumptions and replace them with better ones. Such a process can be referred to as *"experience formation"*.

However, there are big differences in how quickly and effectively people learn: If you assume that lampposts will dodge you if you run at them energetically, the question arises after how many bumps you want to start questioning the assumption.

However, there are many psychological processes that make such experiential learning difficult or even prevent it: individuals receive negative feedback without learning from it.

Such "mechanisms" are discussed in detail, for example, in the theory of personality disorders and in the theory of self-deception (see Sachse, 2020).

Individuals can form very unfavorable constructions, i.e., models of reality, in their biography and cling to these, despite contradictory information (they do, for example, "more of the same").

30.2 Evaluations

Such assumptions of reality and constructions are then psychologically processed in a very relevant way *"further"*: The person *evaluates* them based on their (implicit and explicit) motives, goals, norms, etc.: A certain assumption (= construction) is thus evaluated as positive, neutral, or negative.

One can and must therefore distinguish *two* processing processes:

1. In the first process, a person forms a model of reality based on data.
2. In the second process, she *evaluates* aspects of the reality model based on motives and norms.

Both processing processes can be unfavorable (lead to high costs) or favorable, and both can and should be clearly distinguished in the therapy process.

In an *evaluation*, the person compares constructions and assumptions (from their point of view: "facts") with their motives, goals, desires, and then evaluates them as *personally* positive, neutral, or negative.

> Therefore, it is essential to distinguish between constructions and their evaluations: Constructions are formed by interpretations of "data". Evaluations are formed by evaluating these constructions through motives, goals, etc.

A person, for example, has developed a construction about herself, e.g., that she cannot do Y. This construction can in itself already be more or less valid or invalid, and therefore can (and should) be disputed and tested as such.

But that's not the whole story: The person can now have a norm that one should be able to do Y and that one is worthless if not. Or she assumes that the lack of Y leads to her not being able to achieve certain goals. In such cases, she *evaluates* the lack of Y as (more or less) *negative*.

> Thus, she draws *two* conclusions:
>
> - She forms the construction: "I am a failure".
> - And she makes the evaluation: "Therefore, I am worthless, shit" etc.
>
> One must see that these are *two processes* that can not only be distinguished but also should be distinguished.

Such evaluations, as it becomes clear here, are a *second construction process:*

- In the first construction, a model of reality is developed.
- In the second construction, the assumptions of reality are evaluated based on norms, goals, etc.

Thus, both reality constructions and evaluations are

- psychologically just *constructions,*
- which can be formed psychologically by many factors,
- which are more or less valid, justified, or sensible,

- and which can in any case be questioned psychotherapeutically,
- and should also be questioned, or, if they cause problems, must be questioned.

Clients may now tend not to make this distinction: For them, "failure" and "shit" are one: One necessarily follows from the other.

However, clients should recognize that both processes can and should be considered independently of each other.

For example, I can come to the conclusion that I can't do something. But with that, I can also quite possibly come to the conclusion that that's *okay*, that I can accept it.

Therefore, clients should learn in therapy to separate reality constructions and evaluations. And therefore, the therapist should make it clear that these are *two* processes that can be considered and disputed independently of each other.

A significant therapeutic consequence is that constructions of reality and evaluations can be worked on, disputed, and changed independently of each other.

The therapist and client may come to the conclusion that a reality construction can or must be seen as valid: A client really does not have certain abilities. However, one can still work on the evaluation ("therefore I am worthless") and significantly change *this*.

Reality constructions and evaluations must also be approached differently in therapy (cf. Sachse, 2003). If a therapist does not separate these aspects, he misses out on essential therapeutic approaches.

However, it is also essential for a therapy concept to make such a distinction: If one only speaks of "beliefs", there is a risk of mixing these two aspects. And such mixtures "obscure" the problem: A separation, on the other hand, creates many therapeutic approaches.

Such confusions can also be found in many terms. This will be illustrated here using the example of "guilt": If you analyze the term "guilt", it becomes clear that it is composed of a reality construction and an evaluation.

The reality construction implies

- the assumption that one's own actions have caused a certain effect, i.e.
- in a psychological sense, being responsible for the effect oneself.

The evaluation aspect implies even more, namely

- that my actions contradict a norm or a moral standard
- and/or that the effect should not have occurred based on such standards
- and that the person considers this standard to be binding
- and thus concludes that their actions or even they as a person are reprehensible, i.e. "guilty".

Both aspects can and should now be disputed independently of each other.

So "responsibility" implies

- that the person could have acted differently,
- that they had the effect under control,
- that they should have anticipated the result,
- that they could therefore have made a different decision, etc.

All these aspects can be disputed in the process. If you do this, you often recognize misconceptions here: The client may not have had the effect under control, they may not have been able to anticipate the result, they may not have been able to act differently in a meaningful way.

This psychologically inevitably results in the client not having any responsibility for the result. And: If they have no responsibility, they cannot be "guilty".

But even if the analysis concludes that the client had responsibility and could have acted differently, this does not necessarily have to result in "guilt". Because one can now certainly dispute the moral standards, their validity, their consequences, etc.

And even if this should lead to the conclusion that one has violated standards that one wants to recognize as binding, one can dispute whether or under what conditions one can "forgive oneself".

Thus, the "dissolution" of the implication structure of "guilt" opens up many different therapeutic approaches. So here too, it is again about the therapist understanding the client very precisely, that he understands what a client "means", which concepts he includes (we call this "implication structure") and clarifies and disputes the individual aspects.

References

Baumann, P. (2015). *Erkenntnistheorie*. Metzler.

Ernst, G. (2016). *Einführung in die Erkenntnistheorie*. Wissenschaftliche Buchgesellschaft.

Förstl, H. (2007). *Theory of Mind – Neurobiologie und Psychologie sozialen Verhaltens*. Springer.

Gabriel, M. (2016). *Die Erkenntnis der Welt – Eine Einführung in die Erkenntnistheorie*. Verlag Karl Alber.

Grundmann, T. (2017). *Analytische Einführung in die Erkenntnistheorie*. De Gruyter.

Sachse, R. (2003). *Klärungsorientierte Psychotherapie*. Hogrefe.

Sachse, R. (2020). *Die Psychologie der Selbsttäuschung*. Springer.

31

Alienation

"Alienation" means that a person is no longer able to perceive and represent their own motives. This impairs their satisfaction and well-being and leads to massive problems. Therapists should recognize and therapeutically address alienation.

In motivational psychology, there is a distinction that is also of extreme importance psychotherapeutically: The distinction between explicit and implicit motives (cf. Brunstein, 2006, 2010; Brunstein & Hoyer, 2002; McClelland, 1958, 1987; Schultheiss & Brunstein, 1999, 2001).

Implicit motives are to be seen as the more central, significantly meaningful for a person.

These are motives,

- that are the "actual" fundamental motives of a person,
- whose satisfaction (and *only* their satisfaction!) creates satisfaction.

Implicit motives probably form early in the biography through corresponding affective experiences (McClelland, 1958, 1987).

Implicit motives are strongly affective and very little cognitive: A person "feels" more what they want than they "think" it.

Therefore, implicit motives are central to a person, and their satisfaction is essential to create satisfaction and "meaningfulness" (cf. Brunstein et al., 1995, 1998, 1999, 2007; Brunstein & Maier, 1996, 2002).

R. Sachse, *Basic Psychological Insights for Psychotherapy*,
https://doi.org/10.1007/978-3-662-69780-1_31

However, they are difficult for a person to access because they cannot be "simply cognitively retrieved".

Later, so-called *explicit motives* form, mainly as an internalization of social expectations. A person develops goals here, not because they are *important to them*, but because, for example, their father has defined them as important: Such explicit goals often have the character of *norms*. These explicit motives are strongly cognitive and usually easily accessible to a person: They can therefore easily orient themselves by them (cf. Schultheiss & Brunstein, 1999, 2001).

Explicit motives often contain only small parts of the implicit motives: If a person then follows explicit motives to a high degree, they "live past their motives".

The satisfaction of implicit motives has serious psychological consequences:

- It creates *satisfaction* (and only the satisfaction of *implicit* motives creates satisfaction),
- it generates psychological well-being,
- it creates a sense of meaningfulness, of meaningful and fulfilled life.

If a person does not satisfy these motives over a long period of time, the result is

- *dissatisfaction,* which accumulates and leads to aversive affects, restlessness, etc.,
- psychological tension and discomfort,
- the *feeling of lack of meaningfulness,*
- possibly psychosomatic and depressive developments (cf. Kuhl & Kaschel, 2004).

Therefore, it is of very great *importance* for a person to recognize their own implicit motives, to know them and to take them into account in their own actions, so that there is a chance to satisfy them.

Unfortunately, implicit motives are hardly cognitive, but function according to an affective processing system (Sachse & Langens, 2014).

Therefore, implicit motives can neither be captured by asking questions nor by questionnaires, and the person themselves cannot simply "ask" what they want: They must rather follow so-called "affective indicators" to find out (cf. Sachse & Langens, 2014).

Such "affective indicators" are

- *moods,* which may persist for a long time,
- *physical reactions,* of which the person knows *that* they mean something, but often not *what* they mean,
- *daydreams and fantasies,*
- (in a complex way) *dreams.*

All these indicators

- are not easy to recognize,
- can be easily ignored,
- can only be recognized if a person takes them seriously and pays attention to them,
- are not easily understood.

This is mainly because affective processes are not very cognitive, *but understanding always implies a cognitive interpretation,* a person only understands such indicators and thus the information that the system provides about implicit motives, *if they manage to "translate" affective meanings into cognitive meanings!*

However, this is very difficult, but some people manage to do it to a high degree (never completely), while others manage it poorly or not at all.

If successful, the person has *a good cognitive representation of their motives,* i.e., valid knowledge about what they want, what is good for them, what satisfies them *and* also about what they *do not want,* what is not good for them and what makes them dissatisfied.

Based on this knowledge, *the person can then make decisions* and carry out actions that are highly likely to satisfy the implicit motives. They then live "in harmony with their motive system".

However, there are also people, including many clients, who *have poor or no access to their implicit motive system.* Kuhl and Beckmann refer to this as *Alienation,* i.e., a *estrangement* from their own motive system (cf. Kuhl & Beckmann, 1994a, b; see also: Beckmann, 1997, 2006; Kuhl & Kaschel, 2004).

People with high Alienation...

- do not know what satisfies them and what does not,
- therefore orient themselves towards so-called "explicit motives", which are often not compatible with the implicit motives,
- thus realize actions that do not satisfy their implicit motives, sometimes even massively frustrate them,
- thus live "past their motives" with all the consequences described.

From these considerations result *therapeutic consequences:*

1. Since Alienation is a relevant problem for many clients and thus leads to strongly unfavorable consequences, therapists should always pay attention to signs of Alienation in the process.
2. If Alienation is present, it should be therapeutically addressed. There are specific therapeutic strategies for this (cf. Sachse, 2022).
3. A client who comes to therapy and is thus motivated for therapy is so because they recognize the *costs* of their system and do not want these.
4. From costs arise the first, immediate therapy goals, namely *cost reduction.* These are avoidance goals (C-). Nevertheless, therapists should always start with this, as clients have access to it and can thus take a first step towards *motivation for change.*
5. In the long run, it is important to achieve a motivation for change.
6. While avoidance goals are initially of great importance for this, in the long term a client should pursue *approach goals,* i.e., goals that correspond to their implicit motive system.
7. *This is logically only possible when and only when a client has access to this motivation system.*
8. People who show a high degree of Alienation at the beginning of therapy, however, do not meet this requirement *at all.*

If one takes the concept of Alienation seriously, this means that many clients at the beginning of therapy either cannot define positive goals at all, or, if they are supposed to, define goals from the explicit motive system. If the client's access to their implicit motives improves during the course of therapy, most of these goals must be reformulated.

However, this raises the question of whether it is even sensible to determine positive goals at the start of therapy, and this also massively questions the sense of "goal-attainment-scaling" (cf. Heavlin et al., 1982; Ottenbacher & Cusick, 1990; Smith, 1976; Steinbook et al., 1977).

Undoubtedly, the development of positive goals is very essential from a motivational theory perspective. However, such goals should sensibly be determined *only in the course of the process* when the client's alienation has decreased.

And even then, a verbal, cognitive clarification is by no means sufficient, but imaginative techniques must be used (Bengler, 2021; Kirn et al., 2015).

References

Beckmann, J. (1997). *Alienation and Conformity.* Max-Planck-Institut für psychologische Forschung.

Beckmann, J. (2006). Konsequenzen der Entfremdung vom Selbst. In R. Sachse & P. Schlebusch (Eds.), *Perspektiven Klärungsorientierter Psychotherapie* (pp. 46–59). Pabst.

Bengler, S. (2021). *Praxisbuch Imaginative Techniken in der Psychotherapie: Grundlagen, Techniken und Anwendung.* Springer.

Brunstein, J. C. (2006). Implizite und explizite Motive. In J. Heckhausen & H. Heckhausen (Eds.), *Motivation und Handeln* (pp. 303–329). Springer.

Brunstein, J. C. (2010). Implicit motives and explicit goals: The role of motivational congruence in emotional well-being. In O. C. Schultheiß & J. C. Brunstein (Eds.), *Implicit motives* (pp. 347–373). University Press.

Brunstein, J. C., & Hoyer, S. (2002). Implizites versus explizites Leistungsstreben: Befunde zur Unabhängigkeit zweier Motivationssysteme. *Zeitschrift für Pädagogische Psychologie, 16*(1), 51–62.

Brunstein, J. C., Lautenschlager, U., Nawroth, B., Pöhlmann, K., & Schultheiß, O. (1995). Persönliches Anliegen, soziale Motive und emotionales Wohlbefinden. *Zeitschrift für Differentielle und Diagnostische Psychologie, 16,* 1–10.

Brunstein, J. C., & Maier, G. W. (1996). Persönliche Ziele: Ein Überblick zum Stand der Forschung. *Psychologische Rundschau, 47,* 146–160.

Brunstein, J. C., & Maier, G. W. (2002). Das Streben nach persönlichen Zielen: Emotionales Wohlbefinden und proaktive Entwicklung über die Lebensspanne. In G. Jüttemann & H. Thomae (Eds.), *Persönlichkeit und Entwicklung* (pp. 157–189). Beltz.

Brunstein, J. C., Maier, G. W., & Dargel, A. (2007). Persönliche Ziele und Lebenspläne: Subjektives Wohlbefinden und proactive Entwicklung im Lebenslauf. In J. Brandtstädter & U. Lindenberger (Eds.), *Entwicklungspsychologie der Lebensspanne: Ein Lehrbuch* (pp. 270–304).

Brunstein, J. C., Maier, G. W., & Schultheiß, O. C. (1999). Motivation und Persönlichkeit: Von der Analyse von Teilsystemen zur Analyse ihrer Interaktion.

In M. Jerusalem & R. Pekrun (Eds.), *Emotion, Motivation und Leistung* (pp. 147–167). Hogrefe.

Brunstein, J. C., Schultheiß, O. C., & Grässmann, R. (1998). Personal goals and emotional well-being: The moderating role of motive dispositions. *Journal of Personality and Social Psychology, 75*, 494–508.

Heavlin, W. D., Lee-Merrow, S. W., & Lewis, V. M. (1982). The psychometric foundations of goal attainment scaling. *Community Mental Health Journal, 18*(3), 230–241.

Kirn, T., Echelmeyer, L., & Engberding, M. (2015). *Imagination in der Verhaltenstherapie*. Springer.

Kuhl, J., & Beckmann, J. (1994a). Alienation: Ignoring one's preferences. In J. Kuhl & J. Beckmann (Eds.), *Volition and Personality: Action versus state orientation* (pp. 375–390). Hogrefe.

Kuhl, J., & Beckmann, J. (1994b). *Volition and Personality: Action versus state orientation*. Hogrefe & Huber.

Kuhl, J., & Kaschel, R. (2004). Entfremdung als Krankheitsursache: Selbstregulation von Affekten und integrative Kompetenz. *Psychologische Rundschau, 55*(2), 61–71.

McClelland, D. C. (1958). Methods of measuring human motivation. In J. W. Atkinson (Ed.), *Motives in fantasy, action, and society* (pp. 7–42). Van Nostrand.

McClelland, D. C. (1987). *Human motivation*. Cambridge University Press.

Ottenbacher, K. J., & Cusick, A. (1990). Goal attainment scaling as a method of clinical service evaluation. *The American Journal of Occupational Therapy, 44*(6), 519–525.

Sachse, R. (2022). *Komplexität in der Psychotherapie*. Hogrefe.

Sachse, R., & Langens, T. A. (2014). Bedeutung von Affekten. In R. Sachse & T. A. Langens (Eds.), *Emotionen und Affekte in der Psychotherapie* (pp. 34–46). Hogrefe.

Schultheiß, O. C., & Brunstein, J. C. (1999). Goal imagery: Bridging the gap between implicit motives and explicit goals. *Journal of Personality, 67*(1), 1–38.

Schultheiß, O. C., & Brunstein, J. C. (2001). Assessment of implicit motives with a research version of the TAT: Picture profiles, gender differences and relations to other personality measures. *Journal of Personality Assessment, 77*(1), 71–86.

Smith, D. L. (1976). Goal attainment scaling as an adjunct to counseling. *Journal of Counseling Psychology, 23*(1), 22–27.

Steinbook, R. M., Jacobson, A. F., & Mosher, J. C. (1977). The goal-attainment scale: An instructional guide for the delivery of social reinforcement. *Archives of General Psychiatry, 34*(8), 923–926.

32

Self-Regulation

"Self-regulation" means that a person can reconcile the demands of reality and their motivational system. Self-regulation can be disrupted for many psychological reasons, and therapists should analyze this and restore such regulation.

Good self-regulation can be seen as an important aspect that significantly determines the quality of life of individuals. Poor self-regulation leads to (massive) psychological problems and high individual costs.

Therefore, in psychotherapy, self-regulation can be considered an essential *therapy goal* (Sachse, 2020).

Self-regulation can be defined as a good balance between the demands of reality and the demands of one's own motivational system.

Here, the essential aspects of self-regulation will be addressed.

32.1 Demands of Reality

Clients live (like all people) in a highly complex reality, *which places high demands on them.*

R. Sachse, *Basic Psychological Insights for Psychotherapy*,
https://doi.org/10.1007/978-3-662-69780-1_32

We must be able to meet the demands of our profession, cope with societal and political developments, manage new technical developments, etc. However, our *social context* in particular places high demands on us, and on a daily basis: We must get along with a grumpy boss, deal with highly demanding and manipulative colleagues, endure conflicts, meet expectations, etc.

But our partnership also demands us: A partner has different ideas, goals, and desires than oneself, one must constantly negotiate and find new compromises, one must master interactional crises, etc.

In this context, it can be possible to cope quite well with all these challenges: In this case, one generates "more gains than costs": "Gains" can consist of interaction partners fulfilling one's wishes, taking care of one, taking work off one's hands. But also in being praised and recognized, receiving positive feedback, being appreciated and liked.

Or in being successful, having one's life well under control, being able to influence one's environment, etc.

However, one's own actions in such a context not only yield positive consequences, but also *"costs":* One clashes with interaction partners, has ongoing conflicts, fails to set boundaries, receives negative feedback, accumulates failures, etc.

Overview

This makes it clear that a central life task of a human being obviously consists in coping well with "reality", especially with the social context.

And a person succeeds in this when they achieve *more gains than costs* over a longer period of time.

In complex contexts, which one only has under control to a small extent, it is very likely *not possible to only produce gains:* One will always also incur "costs". Even if one can generally get along well with other people, one will always encounter interaction partners with whom one does not get along and who cause one stress. There will always be people with whom one cannot negotiate and with whom one cannot find compromises. There will always be challenges that one is not up to and that one fails at.

Overview

In the "reality" in which one lives, especially in the social context, one can never only generate gains, i.e., positive consequences. One will always also generate "costs", i.e., experience negative consequences.

One should accept this, and one should prepare for it.

Nevertheless, good coping with reality consists in generating more gains (G) than costs (K): G > K.

Of course, there can always be phases in which the costs outweigh the gains, this is also to be expected. *The goal, however, is that in the long term, averaged over a longer period of time, the gains outweigh.*

Now there are very large differences between individuals in how well they achieve this goal: Some people can apparently *"assess reality well":* They understand, for example, the social rules, can assess interaction partners well, can assess the effects of their actions well, know when they should do something and when not. This maximizes their gains, they show good coping with reality.

Other people, on the other hand, are far less effective: They overestimate their abilities, misjudge social situations, do not understand what interaction partners want and what they despise. As a result, they often act in such a way that they step into "faux pas" or even fall from one bathtub full of fat into the next.

They then generate significantly more costs than gains and thus achieve poor coping with reality.

If they then do not analyze the problem, e.g., because they do not face their mistakes, do not learn from them, do not take responsibility for their actions, always attribute problems to others ("external attribution"), then they cannot learn from mistakes, but they do "more of the same", because they think they can solve the problem by simply increasing the "dose of behavior".

32.2 Demands of the Motivational System

As we have seen, one's own motives also play a crucial role in whether a person can lead a satisfied, fulfilled life or not.

If one analyzes the human psyche more closely, especially with the help of motivational psychology (see above), it becomes clear that a "good adaptation to reality" is not the only central task of a human being.

For a person does not only live in *one* particular type of reality, in and with which they must cope: They also have their own (biological and psychological) conditions.

Thus, people develop so-called "implicit motives" in their biography: These are certain concerns, desires or needs that are very important to a person and that they try to fulfill.

People exhibit different motives, for example:

- the motive for achievement: The person wants to accept challenges, test their own limits, cope with demands, solve tasks, prove their own abilities, etc.
- the motive for connection: The person wants to make contact with others, feel closeness, interact with others, form relationships, etc.
- the motive for recognition: The person wants positive feedback about themselves, their performance, their attractiveness, that they are okay as a person, etc.
- the motive for importance: The person wants feedback that they play a role in the lives of other people, they want to be heard, taken seriously, get attention, etc.

Such motives, it should be understood, play a prominent role in a person's psyche: If a motive is central, then a person wants to satisfy this motive: They develop concrete goals on the way to such satisfaction, act in a way that satisfaction becomes likely, show perseverance, realize a high degree of effort, etc.

Recent motivational psychology has shown that satisfying implicit motives creates a state of *satisfaction*, a positive affective state that feels good to the person and is central to many other psychological processes: It is important for psychological well-being, for recovery, a good immune defense, as protection against stress, etc.

In addition, satisfying implicit motives creates satisfaction and *a subjective feeling of personal meaningfulness, thus conveying the feeling of "life's purpose"*.

Dissatisfaction, especially when it is strong and lasts for a long time, has negative effects:

- It creates a feeling of personal discomfort.
- It creates a feeling of inner restlessness, which can disturb concentration, cause insomnia, etc.
- It creates an internal stress factor, which can severely affect health.
- It can impair the immune defense.
- It leads to a state of meaninglessness, which can be the basis for the development of depression.

Of course, a person can generally *not always be satisfied*: Even if they manage to generally satisfy their needs well, they will always experience phases where they do not succeed well, i.e., they will always have phases of dissatisfaction.

> Therefore, here too, good motive adjustment (to implicit motives) means that a person experiences more satisfaction (S) than dissatisfaction (D) over a longer period of time: S > D.

Just like with reality adjustment, there are also large individual differences here: There are people who achieve a high degree of satisfaction, and those who suffer greatly from dissatisfaction.

A person achieves a high degree of satisfaction when they

- know well which motives are really important to them, i.e., what their (central) implicit motives are,
- have these motives "on their radar" and take them seriously,
- align their actions to satisfy these motives.

On the other hand, if a person does not know their own motives (see "Alienation"), ignores them or does not take them seriously or does not pursue them in their actions, then their chances of satisfying their motives decrease considerably. And thus, the probability increases that they will bring about a state of (permanent) dissatisfaction.

Dissatisfaction accumulates: This means that dissatisfaction grows over time if the person continues to fail to satisfy important implicit motives. Dissatisfaction does not disappear "by itself", e.g., by ignoring it (avoidance preserves a problem)!

The only way to reduce dissatisfaction is to achieve motive satisfaction!

Without such longer-term phases of motive satisfaction, dissatisfaction grows over time: Occasionally short motive satisfactions then temporarily reduce dissatisfaction, but overall dissatisfaction increases.

In such a development, two critical thresholds can be distinguished:

- the perception threshold (PT) and
- the action threshold (AT).

Mild dissatisfaction often goes "unnoticed" by a person: It does not penetrate consciousness. Or the person can ignore it or exclude it from their attention. They can also realize a systematic *self-deception* here (see below).

From a certain intensity onwards, this is hardly or no longer possible: If this *perception threshold* is exceeded, an aversive mental state can no longer be ignored: The person does not necessarily have to understand that it is about "dissatisfaction". However, they clearly notice that "something is not right". They then feel a negative mood, an "inner restlessness" or similar.

Even then, the person does not have to act: They can "endure" the state or try to regulate it. And again, they can realize a systematic self-deception: They can convince themselves that "everything is not so bad", "one can endure it well" or "the state disappears anyway by itself" and similar.

However, if the intensity continues to increase, the *action threshold* is also exceeded. The person then tends to "do something": If they know what the problem is, they can now start working on satisfying a motive and systematically reducing their dissatisfaction.

Often the person does not understand the problem themselves: They do not even know that it is about dissatisfaction, or they do not know what causes it.

In this case, they cannot act purposefully! They then do something: wellness, massages, sports, etc., but notice that this does not work in the long term and then tends to do more of the same. Or they perform even more, even though performance is not the point, as they are not fundamentally performance-motivated. However, this does not satisfy the motive, but rather leads to the person doing even less to satisfy their actual motive: Their actions thus increasingly worsen their condition.

32.3 Self-Regulation: A Balance

From the considerations on reality and motivation adjustment, one can now derive what constitutes the "core" of self-regulation: *Self-regulation means finding a way to balance both demands.*

Self-regulation thus means that a person must find and constantly restore a balance between the demands of reality and the demands of their motive system.

Both reality and motives make almost constant demands: The partner wants something, a work colleague wants a favor, the boss has an order, a friend expects a call, etc.

The demands are often time-limited: I complete an order and it is done. However, some demands extend over long periods of time: My partner expects me to be attentive and understanding, and if I am not, there may be negative consequences. My boss expects me to take care of matters, and if I neglect this, he gets angry. There are sometimes "breaks": times when I don't have to act, but even then I can think about what I have to do or will do tomorrow, what can happen if I make mistakes, etc.

My motives are always active: They do not always make themselves noticeable, but they are always "in the background" and want me to do something that satisfies them.

If I ignore the motives for a long time (which I can usually do), this leads to dissatisfaction, as we have seen. *I cannot ignore my motives for a long time without consequences:* If I do, it will have some kind of negative consequences.

When a situation exists in which one is exposed to two different demands, there are two cases:

- The demands of reality and motives can be *compatible*: They do not "clash" and one can fulfill them both reasonably well.
- However, the demands can also be (more or less) *incompatible*: In order to meet the demands of reality, I have to postpone the satisfaction of motives. Or a motive satisfaction "does not go down well in reality" and generates costs. I cannot fulfill both at the same time—if I fulfill one, the other remains unfulfilled.

And this is the basic dilemma of every person:

- In some (lucky) cases, a person follows the demands of reality and at the same time satisfies important motives. For example, the person's boss can give them a job to do. While they are doing it, they notice that the work is fun: The person finds it challenging, the work is interesting, the person experiences successes, etc.

- Unfortunately, this case does not always occur: It will often be the case that completing a task is not fun at all, that the person finds it "boring", that they would much rather do something completely different.

In such cases

- an action that meets the demands of reality may not satisfy the central motives at all or may even (strongly) frustrate them;
- an action that satisfies a motive can lead to the person having problems with reality.

We all know that this can happen very quickly, e.g.

- you take a break because you feel like it, and get into trouble with the boss,
- you refuse to take on a task from a colleague because you don't feel like it—but this leads to a major conflict,
- you flirt with a colleague because you find her attractive, but she feels harassed by it,
- you have a strong desire to be with your partner, but have to spend time in the office, etc. etc.

However, if this is the case, it follows that *very often the demands of the motive system and the demands of reality are difficult to reconcile:*

- If you strongly focus on meeting reality, you often cope well with it, but unfortunately you neglect your motive system: You then become a highly adapted, successful, but also highly dissatisfied person.
- However, if you decide to follow your motives very often, you can collide massively with reality: You get stress at work, with colleagues, are considered unreliable, unsolidary, etc.

If you follow your own motives very strongly, you quickly generate negative consequences in reality. And this—unfortunately—then also has negative effects on the satisfaction of motives.

This makes it clear that trying to "get the demands under one hat" can lead to many mistakes. Maintaining balance is difficult, but the attempt to decide *only* for one side (and thus create clarity) also does not work.

If you consider the attempt to create a *balance* between the demands of reality and those of the motive system as an essential part of self-regulation, then it becomes apparent from the explanations that *self-regulation is a difficult balancing act that must be performed anew each time.* Self-regulation cannot apparently be viewed as a "static" problem that is solved once and then forgotten. Rather, self-regulation is a constant task that keeps reappearing and needs to be solved anew each time. And it is obviously a difficult task.

Apparently, the task of finding a balance can only be mastered if one can recognize and analyze both demands well: If one has both a good reality model and a good motive representation.

And one must be able to make *decisions* (see above), namely those that can minimize costs and accept that one must always accept costs (possibly over a longer period of time).

One must achieve

- to "serve" both types of demands in the long term, otherwise one gets problems "in the system",
- to decide which demand *should be given priority at the moment*, otherwise one can get massive problems,
- to always give room to the demand that is neglected at the moment,
- to create a *viable compromise* for oneself about when to set which priorities, what one can do without for a while and what one wants to react to immediately, etc.

And one should probably bear in mind that this "internal agreement" is not set in stone: It is always necessary to review it and, if necessary, adapt it to changing conditions.

32.4 Problems With Self-Regulation

Since the task of effective self-regulation is so difficult and many mistakes can be made, relatively many people do not succeed or do not do well in such regulation. There are people who try to create clarity by deciding clearly to primarily adapt to reality and largely ignore their own motives. If they are good at this, they manage reality well: They are successful, solve problems, manage conflicts, meet expectations, etc. That is, they generate significantly more gains than costs in reality.

This creates very basic, very complex and very existentially relevant problems, which can manifest in "symptoms" or not: This makes it clear again that the purpose of therapy cannot consist solely in "symptom reduction"!

An example of such problems are people with pronounced narcissistic personality style: These people primarily want to be successful and thus receive as much recognition as possible, by submitting to existing performance norms. If they have the necessary abilities, they then become (very) successful.

However, since they meet performance *standards* (i.e., extrinsic motives) that do not match their actual motives, they cannot satisfy their motives through their actions. However, they often do not realize this themselves: They think that the more successful they are, the more satisfied they should be. But if "success" is not part of the spectrum of their central motives, they can strive as much as they want: They can be massively successful—but they will still not be satisfied. Since they do not realize this, they usually think that they need to become *even more successful* to finally be satisfied: So they do "more of the same", but this has the effect that they live even more "past their motives", and this *intensifies* their dissatisfaction. In this way, they can easily get caught in a vicious circle (cf. Sachse, 2019).

A very similar problem is created by people with so-called "compulsive personality style": They have many so-called *norms*, i.e., "rules" for themselves, which dictate what they must do, should do, or must not do. As a rule, however, these norms do not correspond to their motives at all: They rather cause the person to largely ignore their motives.

If people follow these norms, they can adapt very well to certain aspects of reality: They are very precise, do exactly what they are told, adhere meticulously to rules and regulations, and thus often meet related expectations 100%.

However, the satisfaction of central motives is completely neglected in such an approach: As a result, people live completely past their motives. They "buy" their high adaptation to reality through complete motive frustration (cf. Sachse, 2019).

Regrettably, however, the opposite of this approach also leads to problems: If a person is extremely "hedonistic" and constantly tries to satisfy their motives, regardless of whether they "clash" with reality, then "the empire of reality strikes back". The person is then usually egocentric, pays little attention to interaction partners, "exploits relationships" etc., which (sooner or later) leads to a (significant) deterioration of relationships.

Such problems are often exhibited by people with a so-called histrionic personality style: These people want a high degree of signals of importance.

They want a lot of attention, always want to be in the spotlight, always want to be seen or heard, etc. And they then tend to enforce such expectations on interaction partners radically: If a partner does not give the person enough attention, especially at a party, they are "snubbed". If he is late once, which the person interprets as a sign of "he ignores my needs", "hell breaks loose" etc. (cf. Sachse, 2002).

The goal of all these approaches is to always and unrestrictedly receive attention, i.e., signals of importance, from everyone: The goal is thus to ensure an extremely high satisfaction of a motive.

Regrettably, such actions usually do not go down well with interaction partners: They feel exploited, manipulated, get little in return for their actions, feel strongly devalued and criticized, and eventually have "had enough". And when this state occurs, the person's actions have the opposite effect: The interaction partners are no longer turned towards them, but are annoyed, they break off contacts etc.

Thus, the person usually achieves exactly the opposite of what they want: Everyone "terminates the relationship" and they then get exactly what they centrally want—namely importance—not at all.

In such cases, it would be important to restore an "inner balance":

- Of course, one may try to be very successful, but it is sensible to always look at what is important to oneself, and to allocate time and resources for the satisfaction of motives, even if this sometimes means having to postpone the pursuit of "success goals".
- Of course, it's okay to want attention: But if you want that in a relationship, then you have to create "balance" in the relationship: You also have to take care of satisfying the needs of the interaction partner, even if this sometimes means having to postpone the satisfaction of your own motives.

Therapeutic consequences of such considerations are:

- Therapists should not only focus on "symptoms" in the process.
- They should always view the psychological problems of clients more complexly.
- Some problems of clients are extremely serious and complex.
- And a therapist should then approach such problems systematically,
- which means they also have to prepare for complex and long-term processes (see Fig. 32.1).

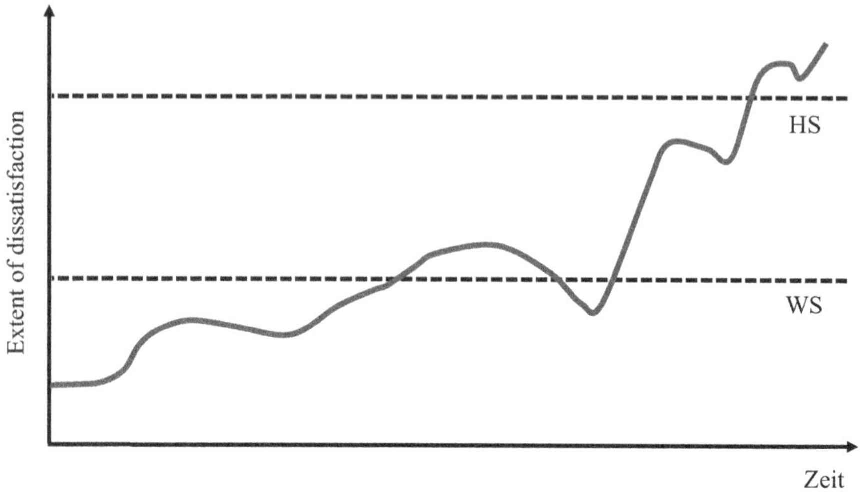

Fig. 32.1 Course of cumulative dissatisfaction. (HS = action threshold WS = perception threshold)

References

Sachse, R. (2002). *Histrionische und narzisstische Persönlichkeitsstörungen*. Hogrefe.
Sachse, R. (2019). *Persönlichkeitsstörungen* (3. ed.). Hogrefe.
Sachse, R. (2020). *Selbstregulation und Selbstkontrolle*. Hogrefe.

33

Self-Deception

A person may want to believe assumptions because they are of personal significance to them. These assumptions can be valid by being compatible with reality, but they can also be (extremely) invalid. In such a case, there is a (systematic) self-deception. Typical self-deceptions are described and their processing is discussed.

As we have seen, for all people, "reality" is a construction: We form a model of reality from observed data and conclusions. And this can be more or less valid.

Psychologically, there can be many reasons for low validity: A particularly important one is *self-deception* (cf. Sachse, 2020).

A *self-deception* occurs when a person

- receives data that suggest a certain conclusion about a certain reality area (e.g., about myself, about relationships, about evolution, etc.), but the person does not want to follow or accept these conclusions due to motives, norms, fears, etc.,
- wants to draw a different conclusion due to these motives, etc., which, however, contradicts the conclusion suggested by the data,
- and then decides to *believe* the conclusion she prefers, i.e., to consider it personally valid and valid (even though it is not),
- and uses cognitive strategies to devalue, discredit, define as untrue or incorrect the conclusions not accepted.

R. Sachse, *Basic Psychological Insights for Psychotherapy*,
https://doi.org/10.1007/978-3-662-69780-1_33

Self-deception thus occurs when the person believes something for which there is no supporting data, or even something that contradicts (well) validated data,

Sachse (2020) has shown that one can (roughly) distinguish five types of *belief*:

1. The person believes conclusions or constructions that are very well validated, for which there are (very) good empirical proofs, i.e., scientifically based theories, etc. Then belief and data (or conclusions from data) do not contradict: This is *not* a case of self-deception.
2. The person believes constructions based on "everyday evidences": on conclusions, therefore, that have been tested in everyday life and have proven themselves. These conclusions do not have the same degree of validity as scientific statements. Nevertheless, they are also *"empirically tested,"* albeit in a possibly unsystematic way. In this case, one cannot speak of self-deception.
3. The person believes constructions that are neither confirmed nor falsified by scientific or everyday empiricism: She thus believes assumptions without any empirical basis. In this case, one should already speak of self-deception, because the person knows that her assumptions are not substantiated, but still holds on to them because they are personally important to her.
4. The person believes constructions that *contradict* everyday empiricism: She thus believes assumptions *against* which empirical evidences speak. This is a significantly higher degree of self-deception, as the person may constantly be confronted with data that refute her assumptions. In this case, she needs cognitive strategies to support and protect her assumptions against evidences.
   She can, for example, assume/assert,
   - the data are not valid,
   - have been misinterpreted,
   - other important information has been overlooked,
   - the data are (basically) not relevant, etc.
5. The person can also believe constructions that contradict (very) well validated scientific theories. This can be considered the most massive degree of self-deception. In such a case, the person needs many, very pronounced or "crass" cognitive strategies to maintain an assumption despite the counter-evidences.

An example of "Belief 1" is when a person believes a scientifically based theory, e.g., that quantum theory or the theory of evolution are correct: These theories are ultimately not "true", but they are extremely well substantiated.

An example of "Belief 2" is when a person considers herself intelligent and many (everyday) data prove this: She has passed exams well, solved problems effectively, received positive feedback, etc.

An example of "Belief 3" is, for example, when a person believes in a supernatural existence: This assumption can neither be proven nor falsified.

An example of "Belief 4" occurs when a person considers herself highly intelligent, although she has failed important exams, dropped out of school, was not successful in many activities, etc.

And an example of "Belief 5" is when a person defines a well-founded scientific theory as "untrue", "false", "not proven", etc.

The latter occurs with the so-called "creationists" when they describe the theory of evolution (which can be considered one of the best-evaluated theories ever) as incorrect (cf. Beck, 1979; Bliss, 1978; Braun-Urban, 1982; Godfrey, 1983; Illies, 1980; Parker, 1980; Riegle, 1974).

Psychologically, it must be assumed that not every type of self-deception generates negative effects, i.e., costs.

There are also so-called "positive illusions" (Försterling & Morgenstern, 2006), which have a rather favorable psychological effect, e.g., a person's assumption that they have a lot of control over their life (much more than may actually be the case). This self-deception is very common *and* it is apparently essential for good psychological functioning.

There are also *neutral self-deceptions,* i.e., those that neither positively nor negatively affect a person. Whether the person believes something specific or not has no significant influence on their life.

However, many self-deceptions have negative or even extremely negative effects: For example, if I believe that I have outstanding qualifications as a driver, but in reality only have an average level of competence, I behave very riskily in traffic. I believe that I can easily drive into a construction site at 160 km/h; however, the reality may be that I end up on a guardrail or even endanger or kill other road users.

Therapeutically, it is very important that a client recognizes and modifies self-deceptions that lead to (strongly) negative effects.

To do this, a client must recognize such self-deceptions and understand the costs they entail.

The therapist should confront the client so that they can recognize

- that they are making assumptions that do not match reasoned conclusions,
- that lead to (strongly) negative consequences,
- why they are making these assumptions, i.e., why they want to believe them,
- that they should question and dispute these reasons.

However, a therapist should not overdo it here: A client should "indulge" in a certain amount of self-deception, as long as the costs for it remain within acceptable limits.

However, if as a client I no longer want to bear certain costs, I will have no choice but to deal with my "belief".

References

Beck, H. W. (1979). *Biologie und Weltanschauung*. Hänssler.

Bliss, R. (1978). *Origins – Two Modells – Evolution, Creation*. San Diego.

Braun-Urban, H. (1982). *Der Mensch stammt nicht vom Affen ab*. Schulz.

Försterling, F., & Morgenstern, M. (2006). Positive Illusionen. In H.-W. Bierhoff & D. Frey (Eds.), *Handbuch der Sozialpsychologie und Kommunikationspsychologie* (pp. 363–372). Hogrefe.

Godfrey, L. R. (1983). *Scientists Confront Creationism*. W.W. Norton.

Illies, J. (1980). *Schöpfung oder Evolution*. Interfrom.

Parker, G. (1980). *Creation – The facts of life*. Creation Life Publishers.

Riegle, D. (1974). *Evolution – Eine Irrlehre?* Hermann Schulte.

Sachse, R. (2020). *Die Psychologie der Selbsttäuschung*. Springer.

34

Therapeutic Rules

Both from the results of process research and from theoretical considerations, therapeutic rules can be derived for therapists, which a therapist can use as a guide.

As a summary of the book, I would like to conclude my remarks in some *therapeutic rules* that therapists can use as a guide.

I would like to keep the explanations brief, as the reasons for this have already been given in detail in the previous text.

1. **Always design the therapy and the therapy process to suit the client!** Pay attention to what a client wants and needs, and note that this may only become clear during the course of therapy. Consider the high heterogeneity and therefore *adapt to this particular client!*
2. **Create a client model!** Create a model (or case concept) about the client as a basis for all therapeutic decisions.
3. **Always consider diagnoses and models as hypotheses!** Diagnoses and models can be well validated, but they always remain hypotheses.

And these

- must always be checked again,
- must be supplemented, elaborated, modified and possibly discarded.

R. Sachse, *Basic Psychological Insights for Psychotherapy*,
https://doi.org/10.1007/978-3-662-69780-1_34

4. **Formulate process goals!** Analyze the client process and develop process goals from the model. Try to pursue these consistently and "straight".
5. **Derive interventions and strategies from the client model!** Interventions and strategies should always be derived from the client model, both from the status model and from the process model.
6. **Always design interventions according to certain rules!** Interventions should always be designed according to certain rules, so for example, they should be short, concise, and easy to understand.
7. **Always pay attention to the client process!** The client process is highly variable, and anything can happen: A therapist should always know *what* is happening right now.
8. **Control the client process!** A therapist should control the client process to a high degree, so "take process responsibility".
9. **Pay attention to changes in the topic!** In the process, new, highly relevant content can emerge, which a therapist should perceive and react to.
10. **React flexibly!** As long as a therapist can control a process stringently, he should do so. However, he should be able to react flexibly to new, relevant content.
11. **Pay attention to the effects of your interventions!** A therapist should always pay attention to how his intervention works, whether the client implements it or not, and he should react flexibly to it.
12. **On the edge of the possible!** Control the client process in such a way that a client is challenged, but not overwhelmed.

The manufacturer's authorised representative in the EU is Springer Nature Customer Service Centre GmbH, Europaplatz 3, 69115 Heidelberg, Germany. If you have any concerns regarding our products, please contact ProductSafety@springernature.com

Printed and bound by CPI Group (UK) Ltd, Croydon, CR0 4YY
28/09/2026
02224082-0004